Handbook of Endobronchial Ultrasound

Madhusmita Mohanty Mohapatra
Pratap Upadhya

Handbook of Endobronchial Ultrasound

Diagnosis and Interventions

Springer

Madhusmita Mohanty Mohapatra
Department of Pulmonary Medicine
Jawaharlal Institute of Postgraduate Medical Education and Research
Puducherry, Pondicherry, India

Pratap Upadhya
Department of Pulmonary Medicine
Jawaharlal Institute of Postgraduate Medical Education and Research
Puducherry, Pondicherry, India

ISBN 978-981-96-0533-0 ISBN 978-981-96-0531-6 (eBook)
https://doi.org/10.1007/978-981-96-0531-6

This Springer imprint is published by the registered company Springer Nature Singapore Pte Ltd.
The registered company address is: 152 Beach Road, #21-01/04 Gateway East, Singapore 189721, Singapore

This handbook is dedicated to the tireless pursuit of knowledge and excellence in the field of endobronchial ultrasound (EBUS) and its applications. To the practitioners, educators, and innovators who have committed themselves to advancing the frontiers of interventional pulmonology, this book is a tribute to your dedication and passion.

Foreword

As we stand at the intersection of medical innovation and diagnostic precision, the emergence of endobronchial ultrasound (EBUS) has ushered in a transformative era within interventional pulmonology. It is with great pleasure and anticipation that I introduce this comprehensive handbook, crafted with meticulous attention to detail, to guide both novice and seasoned practitioners in the realm of endobronchial ultrasounds and its applications.

The exponential growth in our understanding of pulmonary and mediastinal pathology owes much to the ground-breaking advancements encapsulated within these pages. Driven by an unwavering commitment to excellence, the authors have distilled their collective expertise into a concise yet thorough manual, offering a roadmap through the intricate landscape of EBUS-related theory and technicality.

This handbook navigates the reader through the fundamental aspects of EBUS, from the intricacies of anatomy and lymph node station identification to the details of instrumentation and patient preparation. The inclusion of vital information on indications, contraindications, technical aspects of scope insertion, manipulation, and sampling, as well as insights into potential complications, serves as a compass for practitioners seeking mastery in the field.

In the rapidly evolving era of medical science, staying abreast of the latest guidelines is imperative. This handbook not only encapsulates the current standards but also provides a glimpse into the future of EBUS, showcasing its pivotal role in the detection of early cancer and the staging of pulmonary conditions.

It is evident that this handbook is a compilation of facts for those who tirelessly strive to enhance the capabilities of interventional pulmonology. To the practitioners, educators, and researchers who have contributed to this work; your collective efforts have yielded a valuable resource that will undoubtedly enrich the learning journey of individuals across diverse medical backgrounds.

In closing, this foreword serves as an invitation to embark on a journey through the intricacies of EBUS—a journey that promises to expand your knowledge, sharpen your skills, and contribute to the ongoing narrative of progress in pulmonary medicine. May this handbook illuminate the path of practitioners ensuring that the benefits of EBUS reach every corner of patient care.

Professor and Head, Department of Pulmonary Medicine
JIPMER, Puducherry, India

Saka Vinod Kumar

Preface

In crafting this inaugural edition of our handbook on endobronchial ultrasound, our aim has been to distil the complexities of EBUS and its applications into a handbook for easy understanding. With a focus on anatomy, instrumentation, and the latest guidelines, this book endeavours to be an indispensable resource for both novices and seasoned practitioners in the realm of interventional pulmonology. As we navigate the intricate landscape of EBUS, I am hopeful that this handbook will serve as a valuable companion, providing practical insights and fostering a deeper understanding of these innovative diagnostic procedures. It is my sincere wish that this resource proves to be not only informative but also instrumental in enhancing the skills and knowledge of trainees and practitioners in the dynamic field of interventional pulmonology.

Puducherry, India Madhusmita Mohanty Mohapatra

Acknowledgements

The creation of this handbook has been a collaborative endeavour, and I extend my deepest gratitude for the blessings of almighty, teachers, and my dear parents. I am grateful to my patients and residents who inspired me to improve my understanding of the subject. My heartfelt thanks to my family for their wholehearted support and encouragement. My appreciation goes to Jagjeet Kaur Saini (Senior Editor) and Chihiro Haraguchi (Senior Editorial Assistant), at Springer Nature for their support, guidance, and commitment to bringing this work to fruition. I would also like to extend my gratitude to my colleagues specially Dr Harshith R Rao, Dr Debasis Gocchait and Dr Karthik Balasoupramaniane for their unwavering support and invaluable contributions in the creation of this book.

Contents

1 Introduction

Modern technology has revolutionized the diagnostic and therapeutic aspect of medical sciences. Traditionally, lung and mediastinal lesions were diagnosed using non-invasive, minimally invasive, and surgical approach. It all started with Gustav Killian in 1876 who removed a pork bone from a farmer's respiratory tract using an esophagoscope. Following his footsteps, Chevalier Jackson laid the milestone for rigid bronchoscope. The era of bronchoscope took a breakthrough when Shigeto Ikeda discovered flexible bronchoscope in the year 1967 which allowed us to investigate the airway mucosa.

Interventional pulmonology reached a new height with the innovation of transbronchial needle aspiration by Ko-Pen Wang for mediastinal lesions and methods of laser photo-resection and stenting by Jean-Francois Dumon. Endobronchial ultrasound-guided transbronchial needle aspiration (EBUS-TBNA) added a new feather to interventional pulmonology by being a novel technique that utilizes integrated conventional bronchoscopy and ultrasound imaging method to get real time sample of lung parenchyma and mediastinal lesions. Pandian et al. were the first to investigate the clinical usefulness of narrow-gauge ultrasonic probe for intravascular ultrasonography. However, Hurter was the first to study the use of EBUS in diagnosis of lung and mediastinal tumors. Peripheral lung nodules can now be assessed with the help of radial EBUS and electromagnetic navigational bronchos-

M. M. Mohapatra, P. Upadhya, *Handbook of Endobronchial Ultrasound*, https://doi.org/10.1007/978-981-96-0531-6_1

copy. Narrow band imaging is an advanced bronchoscopy imaging technique which utilizes green/blue wavelength light to visualize the mucosal surface and capillary patterns of the airway wall. This novel technology helps in early detection of in situ lung cancer.

Future developments in interventional pulmonology are yet to take further turns with introduction of robotic bronchoscopy where the handling and precision for obtaining tissue sample is improvised leading to better and accurate diagnosis. Since, flexible bronchoscope contains minute fibres which needs to be decontaminated to prevent spread of infection, disposable bronchoscopes are being used in infected settings to alienate the difficulty of autoclaving which is a horrendous task to perform in respect to bronchoscope sterilization.

Currently, endoscopic optical coherence tomography is under investigation to obtain detailed information about the layer of bronchial wall under high resolution. With the advent of cryobiospy, electrocautery, argon plasma coagulation, photodynamic therapy, microdebrider bronchoscopy, resector balloon deobstruction, intratumoral chemotherapy and stenting using a rigid or flexible bronchoscope, palliation and management of symptomatic malignant and benign airway lesions to improve quality of life and survival has opened new pathways in management of lung cancer.

This handbook on EBUS is prepared with an intent to provide the beginners with detailed description of the instrument and its related theory and technicality to complement the knowledge and skill required for competency. This handbook will contain information on anatomy and lymph node station, details about instrument, indication and contraindications, patient preparation, technical aspect of scope insertion into airways, manipulation and sampling, complications and guidelines related to EBUS. The aim of this handbook is to enhance the learner's knowledge along the learners curve to make a physician a competent interventionist.

2 Mediastinal Anatomy

It is essential to have knowledge and understanding about the airway anatomy and of the mediastinum before proceeding for endobronchial ultrasound guided transbronchial needle aspiration (EBUS-TBNA). This allows the bronchoscopist to correlate well the radiological findings obtained by computed tomography of thorax with the luminal anatomy before performing bronchioalveolar lavage and biopsy. It is also essential to have an orientation about the ultrasound images of various anatomical structures in the mediastinum and the artifacts that will be encountered during the procedure [1].

The added advantage of EBUS-TBNA over mediastinoscopy is that the targeted lymph node can be selected for biopsy or cytological aspiration based on characteristic ultrasound features. Mediastinoscopy also helps in obtaining biopsy samples from mediastinal lymph node but it requires general anaesthesia and surgeon who are trained in performing emergency thoracotomy and/or sternotomy. Hence, mediastinoscopy has higher interventional risk than EBUS. The ultrasound images of major landmarks like superior vena cava, azygos vein, aorta, heart, thyroid, and other vascular structure should also be clearly recognized and understood for performing EBUS-TBNA.

Many important organs and vessels are found in the mediastinum. It also serves as the conduit and endpoint of all lymphatic drainage. The mediastinum is divided into four compartments:

M. M. Mohapatra, P. Upadhya, *Handbook of Endobronchial Ultrasound*, https://doi.org/10.1007/978-981-96-0531-6_2

superior, anterior, middle, and posterior mediastinum. The disease pattern in all the mediastinum varies considerably and give a clue to the type of disease that confines to a particular mediastinal compartment. All the three mediastinum compartments i.e. anterior, middle and posterior mediastinum contains lymph node while majority of the lymph nodes are observed in the anterio-superior and middle mediastinum. The aetiology of lymphatic pathology varies according to the lymphatic drainage and mediastinal subdivision involved.

The anterior mediastinum is anterior to the pericardium and mainly contains thymus, extrapericardial part of aorta and its branches, the great veins and the lymphatic tissues. The middle mediastinum is a compartment bounded by pericardium anteriorly, the posterior pericardial reflection, the mediastinal pleura, the diaphragm below and the thoracic inlet above. This compartment includes the heart, intrapericardial great vessels, pericardium, trachea and the mediastinal lymph nodes. The posterior compartment extends from the posterior pericardial reflection to the posterior border of the vertebral bodies and from first rib to diaphragm. The great vessels within the mediastinum include aorta, superior venacava, inferior venacava, main pulmonary artery, intrapericardial segments of the trunk of the right and left pulmonary artery, and intrapericardial segments of the superior and inferior right and left pulmonary veins. The mediastinal and thoracic lymph nodes that can be accessed by endoscopy are situated in the anterior, superior and middle compartments which are adjacent to the airways for EBUS TBNA. Furthermore, the posterior mediastinal lymph nodes can be reached through transoesophageal endoscopic ultrasound-guided fine needle aspiration.

Intrathoracic lymph nodes have been mapped into 14 stations according to their proximity of landmarks as observed during mediastinoscopy and thoracotomy for lung cancer. The term station refers to a collection of lymph nodes in a particular anatomical position. The naming convention for mediastinal lymph node employs a combination of anatomical description and numerical system, where "L" represents left and "R" signifies right. Lymph node stations 1–9 correspond to mediastinal nodal groups and are present in the mediastinal pleural reflection. The stations 10–14 representing hilar nodes along with other more peripheral extra mediastinal nodal groups are together located in the visceral pleura. Hence, knowledge of thoracic lymph node is important as it denotes the extent of spread of tumour.

2.1 Lymph Node Stations as Classified by International Association for the Study of Lung Cancer (IASLC) (Fig. 2.1)

Station 1: Station 1 comprises of supraclavicular lymph nodes present in the sternal notch, supraclavicular, and lower cervical regions. This station extends from cricoid cartilage above till the upper margin of the sternal manubrium and clavicle inferiorly. The lymph nodes are designated as right and left i.e. 1R & 1L in relation to the midline of the trachea.

Station 2: Station 2 are the upper paratracheal lymph nodes and present on the lateral wall of the trachea. The upper border of station 2 is delineated by the apex of the ipsilateral lungs and pleural spaces while the lower border on the right side (2R) is where the inferior margin of the left brachiocephalic vein crosses the trachea, while the lower border of station 2 on the left (2L) is the superior border of the aortic arch.

Station 3: The Station 3 lymph nodes are designated as anterior or posterior (A or P). The prevascular lymph nodes called as 3A nodes are located behind the sternum but anterior to the 3superior vena cava and left carotid artery. The prevascular nodes extends to the level of the carina caudally. The retrotracheal lymph nodes (3P) are posterior lymph nodes located posterior to the trachea extending from the apex of the chest to the carina.

Station 4: The lower paratracheal nodes along the distal trachea comprises the Station 4 lymph nodes extending to the level of the carina. They lie posterior to the aortic vasculature, and the lateral wall of the trachea is used to differentiate between 4R and 4L.

Station 5: They are the subarotic lymph nodes and are also known as aortopulmonary (AP) window nodes. They are located lateral to the ligamentum arteriosum, the remnant of the ductus

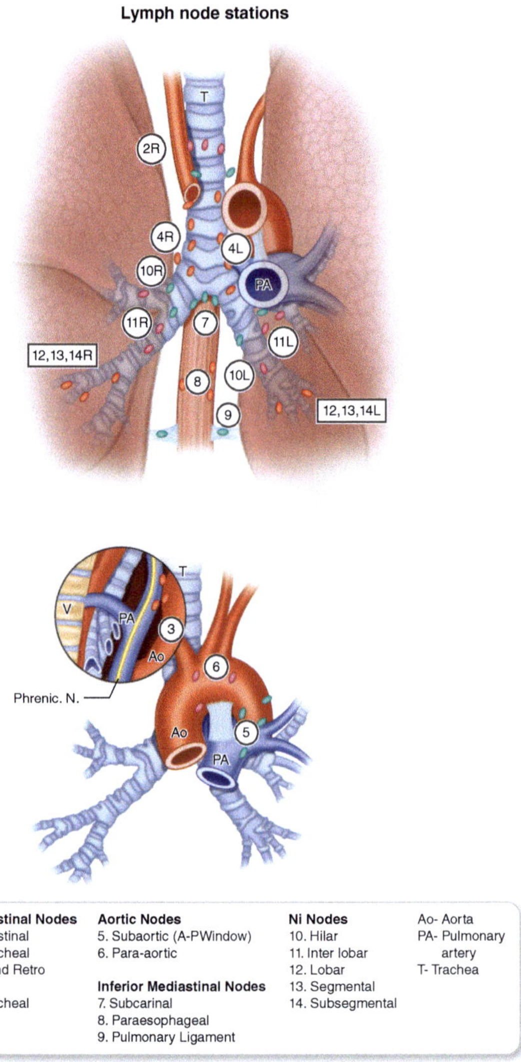

Fig. 2.1 Mediastinal lymph node station as defined by International Association for the Study of Lung Cancer (IASLC). (Photo Courtesy- Dr. Karthik Balasoupramaniane)

arteriosus. They are bounded by lower margin of the aortic arch above and by the superior margin of the left pulmonary artery below.

Station 6: The para-aortic lymph nodes lie on the anterior and lateral aspect of the ascending aorta and aortic arch. The phrenic nerve may be used as a landmark for identifying paraaortic lymph nodes.

Station 7: The subcarinal lymph nodes lie directly below the carina and between the two mainstem bronchi. They are found more caudal to the paraesophageal lymph nodes and are bounded by the distal aspect of the bronchus intermedius and origin of the left lower lobe bronchus.

Station 8: The paraesophageal nodes are the mediastinal lymph nodes found inferior to the subcarinal lymph nodes, along with the anterior or lateral aspects of the esophagus, down to the esophageal hiatus of the diaphragm.

Station 9: The pulmonary ligament nodes are associated with the pulmonary ligaments. These ligaments represent the mediastinal parietal pleural reflections that occur below the right and left pulmonary roots and designated as right and left pulmonary ligament nodes (9R and 9L).

Station 10: These hilar lymph nodes are found along the right and left mainstem bronchi, before they bifurcate, and are designated 10R and 10L, respectively.

Station 11: These interlobar lymph nodes are located between the lobar bronchi, just beyond the bifurcation of each mainstem bronchi.

Stations 12–14: These peripheral nodes are also known as lobar, segmental, and subsegmental lymph nodes, depending on whether they are located along the lobar, segmental, or subsegmental bronchi. These lymph nodes are node frequently and normally encountered.

The IASLC TNM staging (primary tumour-regional lymph node -distant metastasis) for lung cancer in their eighth edition had performed many revisions for the tumour size and metastatic component but there were no distinct changes made in the nodal staging for mediastinal and hilar lymph nodes. This system of classification was made to be adopted for non-small cell lung carcinoma. The small cell lung cancer however does not adopt such system of classification. They follow the conventional system of disease classification as limited type and extensive type [2]. The nodal staging Nx denotes that the regional lymph node cannot be assessed while N0 denotes no nodal spread N1 represents metastasis to ipsilateral intrapulmonary, hilar or peri bronchial lymph nodes. The N3 status in the eighth edition of TNM staging denotes involvement of contralateral mediastinal lymph nodes or supraclavicular lymph nodes or nodes on either side [3].

IASLC TNM lung cancer lymph node staging.

N0	No regional lymph node metastasis
N1	Metastasis in ipsilateral peribronchial and/or perihilar lymph nodes and intrapulmonary nodes, including involvement by direct extension
N2	Metastasis in ipsilateral mediastinal and/or subcarinal lymph nodes
N3	Metastasis in contralateral mediastinal, contralateral hilar, ipsilateral or contralateral scalene, or supraclavicular lymph nodes

Many of the mediastinal nodes are situated in close proximity to the left innominate vein, the anterior surface of the trachea, the circumference of the main bronchi as well as below and to the left of the aortic arch. EBUS TBNA allows for the sampling within a range of 5–7 mm from the airway wall, enabling access to the paratracheal, subcarinal and hilar lymph nodes. This means that both mediastinal and hilar stations can be sampled in a single endoscopic procedure [4]. EBUS TBNA provides the opportunity to diagnose both benign and malignant diseases from hilar and/or mediastinal lymph nodes, including reactive lymphadenopathy, inflammatory diseases, infections and primary or secondary malignancies. Minimally invasive access to these mediastinal lymph nodes is crucial, especially considering that surgical removal is not recommended for patients with non-small cell lung cancer when the tumour effects the central mediastinal lymph nodes [5].

References

1. Becker HD. Bronchoscopy for airway lesions. In: Wang KP, Mehta AC, editors. Flexible bronchoscopy. London: Blackwell Scientific Publications; 1995. p. S.136–59.
2. Edge SB, Compton CC. The American Joint Committee on Cancer: the 7th edition of the AJCC cancer staging manual and the future of TNM. Ann Surg Oncol. 2010;17(6):1471–4. https://doi.org/10.1245/s10434-010-0985-4.
3. Goldstraw P, Chansky K, Crowley J, et al. The IASLC Lung Cancer Staging Project: proposals for revision of the TNM stage groupings in the forthcoming (eighth) edition of the TNM classification for lung cancer. J Thorac Oncol. 2016;11:39.
4. Shirakawa T, Miyazawa T, Becker H. The layer structure of central airways as described by endobronchial ultrasonography (EBUS). J Bronchol. 2008;15(3):129–33. https://doi.org/10.1097/LBR.0b013e31817bd7d9.
5. Wei S, Asamura H, Kawachi R, Sakurai H, Watanabe S. Which is the better prognostic factor for resected non-small cell lung cancer: the number of metastatic lymph nodes or the currently used nodal stage classification? J Thorac Oncol. 2011;6(2):310–8. https://doi.org/10.1097/JTO.0b013e3181ff9b45.

Instrument EBUS Scope

3

The Endobronchial Ultrasound scope consist of a bronchoscopy unit and an ultrasound unit.

Bronchoscopy unit: The bronchoscopy unit is like the normal bronchoscopy unit that has a handle, insertion tube and a flexible tip. The handle consists of a light source, video adaptor, working channel, suction port and angulation control lever (Fig. 3.1).

The length of the scope in total is around 890 mm. The insertion tube has an outer diameter of 6.3 mm and the distal end outer diameter ranges from 6.6 to 6.9 mm. The distal end has objective video lens, light guide lens, ultrasound transducer and instrument channel outlet (Fig. 3.2).

The optical system uses white light and gives a field of view of 80°. The forward oblique view ranges from an angle of 20° to 35° and the depth of field of view varies from 2 to 50 mm. The working channel of a EBUS scope varies from 2.2 to 2.8 mm and the tip can bend upward at an angle ranging from 120° to 160°. The downward movement of the EBUS scope attains a maximum angulation of 70°.

Ultrasound unit: The ultrasound unit consist of a processor and a probe driving unit. The processor is the endoscopic ultrasound center EU-ME2 and EU-ME3 (for Olympus) and it allows to obtain ultrasound images by connecting via probe driving unit MAJ-1720(for Olympus). The ultrasound unit uses ultrasonic waves in the form of echo to generate images (Fig. 3.3).

M. M. Mohapatra, P. Upadhya, *Handbook of Endobronchial Ultrasound*, https://doi.org/10.1007/978-981-96-0531-6_3

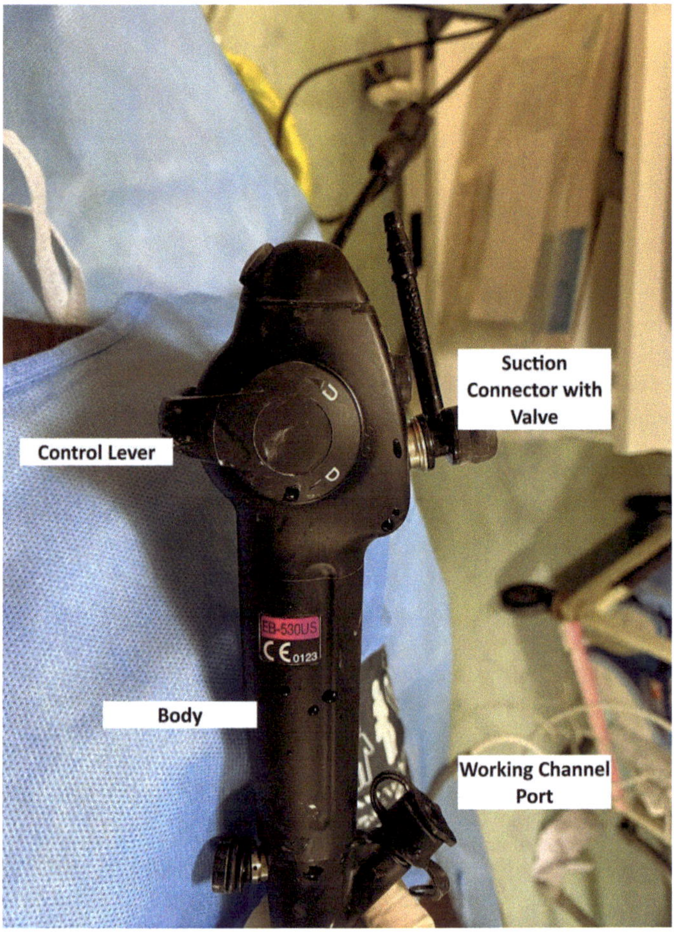

Fig. 3.1 The parts of an endobronchial ultrasound bronchoscope

Smaller waves of echo are transmitted from transducer into the body tissue with different acoustic impedance. Some of these waves are reflected to the transducer and these signals are pro-

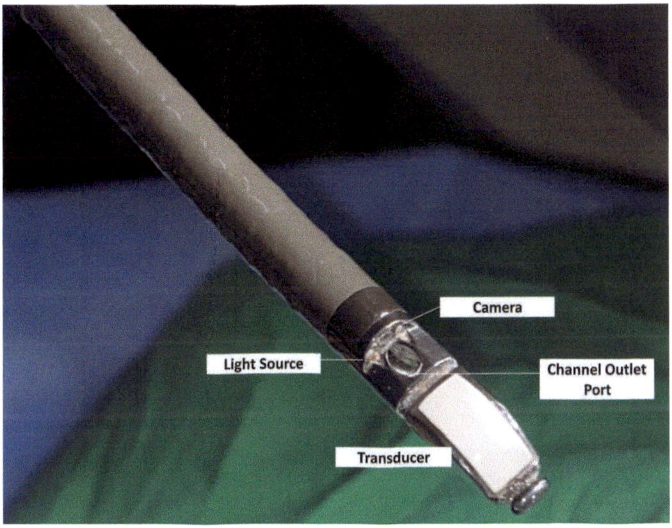

Fig. 3.2 The distal end of convex endobronchial ultrasound bronchoscope with it parts

cessed to form images. The frequency of sound used to identify various tissue structure by ultrasound varies and hence transducers are classified based on the structures that can be identified. Most diagnostic sonography for medical uses has a frequency range of 2–20 MHz. Transducers that identify superficial structures are of high frequencies and have a range of 10–15 MHz and transducers which identifies deeper structure have frequency range of 2–5 MHz.

There are three basic modes that are used in ultrasound to identify various tissue materials. The A mode is amplitude mode, B mode is the brightness mode for visual representation of the echo signals, and M mode is the motion mode for display of echo reflection over time which are commonly used in all basic ultrasound.

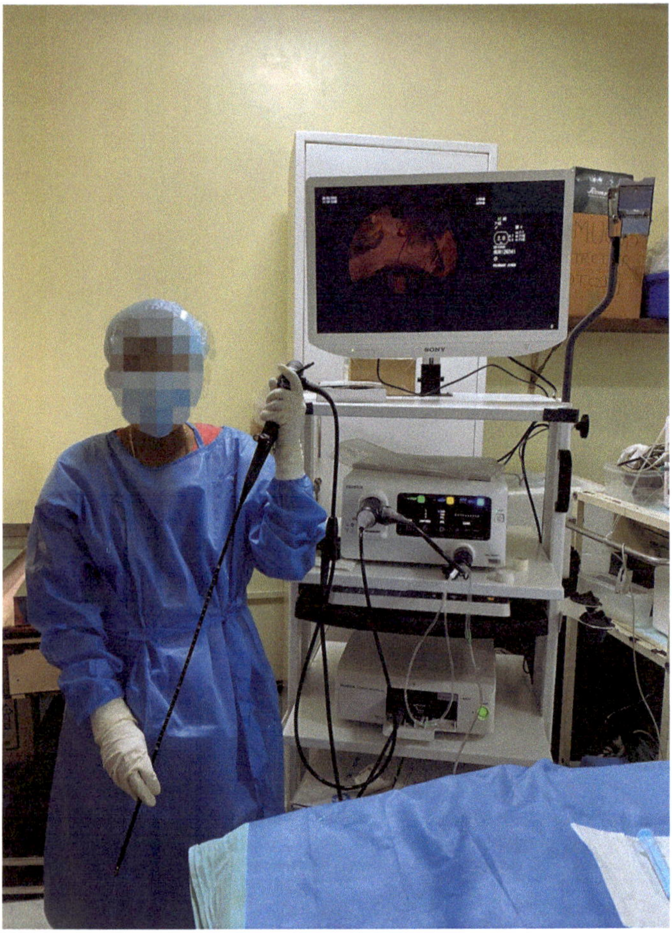

Fig. 3.3 The arrangement showing console along with the ultrasound processor and probe driving unit

3.1 Newer Additions in Ultrasound Component

An important component of newer ultrasound machine is that of tissue harmonics imaging which is also incorporated in EBUS. Tissue harmonic imaging (THI) is a non-linear propagation of ultrasound waves through the tissue where high pressure portion of the wave travels faster than the low-pressure portion thereby causing distortion of the shape of the wave. This dynamic change in the waveform causes formation of harmonics from the tissues. Harmonic waves increase with the depth to a point where a maximum intensity is obtained beyond which it decreases with depth due to attenuation. Therefore, beyond a critical point below the surface harmonic imaging works best. The transducer produces fundamental harmonics with limited reception and hence low noise, wide dynamic range receiver is required to process weak signal. This is done by two methods: (i) harmonic band filtering (ii) pulse phase inversion to remove the fundamental echo and generate only tissue harmonic component for image generation. In today's era, second generation harmonic imaging is being used to acquire a proper image. The advantages of tissue harmonic imaging are that it decreases reverberation artifacts, increases resolution in patients with obesity, increases axial and lateral resolution and gives a clear image of cysts. However, the disadvantage of THI is that it is less sensitive than basic B mode and cannot delineate structures located near the transducer with clarity. Hence, THI works better in addition to B mode but may not be sensitive in differentiating between inflammatory and malignant lymphadenopathy [1]. This system is adapted in endobronchial ultrasound (EBUS) of PENTAX and HITECHI model [2].

Contrast enhanced ultrasound is another technology that is upcoming in endoscopic ultrasound (EUS). It can be of high mechanical index or low mechanical index type. The high mechanical index type can be used in EBUS for staging of mediastinal lymph nodes [3]. The low mechanical index type cannot be incorporated in EBUS due to technical reasons. In this method microbubbles of diameter 2–5 μm made up of gas core and encapsulated by stabilizing shell is used so that when introduced to ultrasound waves it compresses under high pressure and expends in low pressure thereby producing harmonic waves. The harmonic signals are separated from the fundamental echo by phase inversion method. This method can very well differentiate between malignant, normal and inflammatory lymph node. A normal lymph node shows hilar predominant normal vascularity while an inflammatory lymph node has more vascularity without much change in hilar vessel architecture. The lymph node can also be differentiated as benign with contrast enhancement present in the cortex which is homogenous in nature while malignant lymph nodes have peripheral or mixed vascularity with loss of hilar type vascularization [4].

Blood flow in doppler is of various kinds but the doppler used in endobronchial ultrasound includes energy doppler that reflects the intensity of blood flow and colour doppler which reflects direction as well as velocity of blood flow. By convention, blood flow moving towards the transducer is coloured red orange while flow moving away from the transducer is blue coloured. Flow modes used in colour Doppler is known by various names like Fine flow, E-Flow, H-flow and B-flow. In EBUS, currently H-flow and fine flow are being used [5]. It uses a transducer of high frequency (20 Hz) for flow mapping so that small vessels and its distribution can be identified. This will help to avoid vessels during needle aspiration and also prevent dilution of the lymph node aspirate with blood.

3.2 EBUS Probes

There are two types of probes available for EBUS TBNA: linear convex probe and radial probe. The linear probe uses the electronic scanning method where a transducer of 7.5 MHz in curvilinear array is introduced attached to the tip of the bronchoscope. The direction of scanning is the direction in which the bronchoscopy is introduced with an angle of 90° to the bronchoscope. This probe helps in diagnostic aspiration of mediastinal lymph nodes,

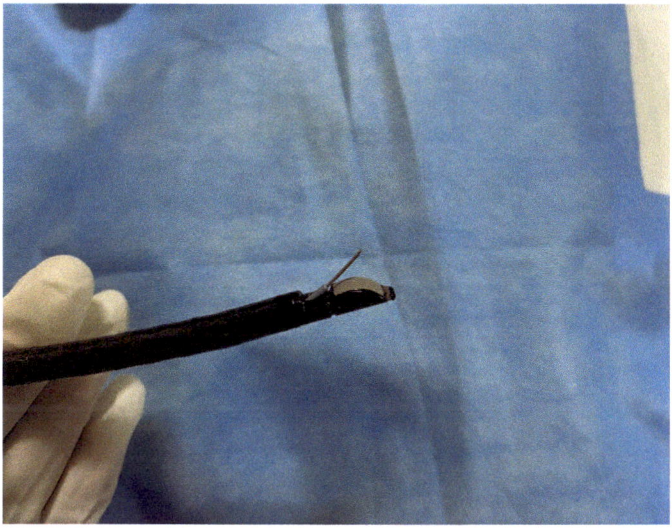

Fig. 3.4 The curvilinear convex or linear probe for endobronchial ultrasound

visualization of mediastinal structures and any mediastinal mass (Fig. 3.4).

The radial probe has transducer for mechanical radial scanning with 360° rotation around the axis of the bronchoscope with a 20Mz frequency which helps in diagnosis of peripheral lung mass. The ultrasound miniprobes used in radial probe use a diameter of <1.7 mm which allows it to pass comfortably through the working channel of the bronchoscope. This helps in inspecting the bronchial wall layers and distinguishing between early and invasive lung cancer. The radial probes inserted into the segmental bronchi shows a snowstorm appearance for normal air-filled alveoli. A dark grey coloured homogenous appearance is seen in the presence of a tumor mass and black colour in the presence of fluid. Usually with radial probe, after identification of a peripheral lesion the probe is removed from the working channel of the bronchoscope and a forceps is introduced to the lesion directly or under fluoroscope guidance for obtaining specimen. Nowadays with new improvised bronchoscope the radial probe is placed in a catheter and passed through the working channel of the bronchoscope. Once the lesion is identified in the periphery, the radial probe is removed and forceps are introduced to obtain the required sample [6].

References

1. Kurimoto N. Endobronchial ultrasonography: an overview. In: Endobronchial ultrasonography. Hoboken: Wiley; 2020. p. 1.
2. Endoscopic Ultrasound | PENTAX Medical (India). https://www.pentax-medical.com/pentax/en/98/17/EB19-J10U-Ultrasound.
3. Dietrich CF. Contrast-enhanced endobronchial ultrasound: potential value of a new method. Endosc Ultrasound. 2017;6(1):43–8. https://doi.org/10.4103/2303-9027.200215.
4. Yusefi H, Helfield B. Ultrasound contrast imaging: fundamentals and emerging technology. Front Phys. 2022;10:791145. https://doi.org/10.3389/fphy.2022.791145.
5. Zhi X, Chen J, Xie F, Sun J, Herth FJF. Diagnostic value of endobronchial ultrasound image features: A specialized review. Endosc Ultrasound. 2021;10(1):3–18. https://doi.org/10.4103/eus.eus_43_20. PMID: 32719201; PMCID: PMC7980684.
6. Zaric B, Eberhardt R, Herth F, et al. Linear and radial endobronchial ultrasound in diagnosis and staging of lung cancer. Expert Rev Med Devices. 2013;10(5):685–95. https://doi.org/10.1586/17434440.2013.827512.

4 Critical Aspects of Ultrasound in EBUS

Understanding the spatial relationship and position of the targeted structure and the bronchial anatomy while performing EBUS procedure requires the consideration of computed tomographic images. Ultrasound images of major vascular structures such as the superior vena cava, aorta, azygos vein and heart should be recognized and colour Doppler method can be used while performing EBUS-TBNA to avoid puncturing of major vascular structures and creating complications. It is to be kept in mind that EBUS cannot access all lymph node stations in the mediastinum. EBUS can access only lymph node stations of 2R, 2L, 4L, 4R, 7, 10L, 10R, 11L, 11R.

The ultrasonographic features of EBUS-TBNA are referred basically to predict whether the lymph node or the lesion are benign or malignant. Most of the interventional pulmonologist use qualitative methods of EBUS to define the characteristics of a benign or malignant lymph node. The most common ultrasound features used in EBUS are gray scale, blood flow Doppler and elastography. The size, shape, margin, echogenicity, central necrosis, and central hilar structure are some of the qualitative ultrasound findings that one has to be oriented with before starting EBUS-TBNA. However, recent studies have shown that a variety of quantitative methods for the three modes are being developed to make a comprehensive scoring system to reduce the subjectivity of the qualitative method [1]. It is to be noted that long axis and

M. M. Mohapatra, P. Upadhya, *Handbook of Endobronchial Ultrasound*, https://doi.org/10.1007/978-981-96-0531-6_4

short axis of the lymph node should be measured in a computed tomography image prior to referring the patient for EBUS so that decision can be made as to whether aspiration from a particular targeted node is possible and whether yield of the sample will be adequate.

4.1 Ultrasound Characteristics of Lymph Nodes in EBUS [1] (Gray Scale Mode)

1. Shape: The long axis and the short axis of the lymph node should also be measured in the ultrasound images. The shape of the lymph node can be round or oval. A node is defined as oval if the ratio between the short axis to long axis is <1.5 and round if the ratio between the short axis to long axis is >1.5.
2. Size: The size of the lymph node determines the yield of the aspirated specimen and hence it is imperative to determine the size of the node both on computed tomography images prior to procedure and via ultrasound imaging during the procedure. The size of the node is usually considered clinically significant when taken in the short axis. The size can be >10 mm or <10 mm in short axis. It is required to differentiate between benign and malignant nodes though it is not meaningful in clinical settings.
3. Margin: The margin of a lymph node is said to be distinct if >50% of the border is clearly visualized and indistinct if <50% of the border is visualized.
4. Echogenicity: The lymph node can have a homogenous or heterogeneous echotexture distribution in relation to the surrounding tissue. The surrounding mediastinal tissues are hyperechoic in nature while the major vascular structures are hypoechoic in nature. Heterogeneity is considered if a node has multiple small areas of different echogenicity excluding major vasculature which are considered as hypoechoic.
5. Central hilar structure: It is defined as a central linear high echogenic area in the lymph node with some blood flow. It can be classified into two types: (1) Central, (2) Eccentric. Central hilar structure sign does not produce characteristic ultrasonic

feature in lymph node if there is infiltration and compression of the node by tumor or necrotic tissue.

6. Coagulation necrosis sign: It is a hypoechoic area in the lymph node without any blood flow. The characteristic ultrasound feature is one low hypoechoic region occupying majority of the lymph node. One study found that the diagnostic accuracy to predict malignant lymph node is 22.1% but there was no statistical significant difference in predicting benign or malignant lymph nodes [2]. The most common cause of coagulation necrosis sign in benign lymph nodes is tuberculosis. This has been confirmed by Dhooria et al. and they found that coagulation necrosis occurs in 26.1% of tuberculosis while occurs in 3.3% of cases of sarcoidosis [3].
7. Colour Power Doppler Index: There are specifically two doppler mode that are used in EBUS.
   i) The energy doppler which indicates intensity and colour doppler which indicates direction of blood flow and are used in early stage. The blood flow image evaluation includes blood flow volume and pattern of vascular distribution.
   ii) The colour power doppler mode can be used to determine the amount of blood flow in the lymph node. The amount of blood flow in the lymph node has been graded from 0 to 3. Grade 0: denotes no blood flow. Grade 1: denotes one or two punctate shaped or small rod shape signal. Grade 2: is one main vessel or few small vessels observed. Grade 3: rich flow of blood within the lymph node. The pattern of vascular distribution in the lymph node is classified based on the blood flow direction signal: (a) avascular, which is absence of blood flow signals within the lymph node (b) hilar, which means the blood flow signal branches radially from the hilum regardless of whether the origin is from central region or from periphery (c) nonhilar, which can be central, capsular and mixed type.
8. Conglomeration of lymph nodes: It is a single lymph node station with multiple enlarged nodes. Few studies have classified nodal conglomeration into two groups: (a) cluster formation (b) matting. Cluster formation occurs when multiple lymph nodes enlarge in size and do not fuse with each other maintain-

ing a well demarked margin. Matting of lymph node occurs when multiple lymph nodes enlarge and fuse together to form a single large lymph node without a well demarked margin and damage of the lymph capsule. Matting often occurs in malignancy when tumor spreads beyond lymph node capsule.

Quantitative assessment of echogenicity in lymph nodes involve use of gray scale texture features. When first order gray scale texture feature is used, it calculates the mean gray value in terms of pixel within the region of interest (ROI) and when second order gray scale features are used, it is assessed based on colour variance within the region of interest which in turn is calculated based on entropy, contrast, correlation, energy and homogeneity.

The presence of round shape, size >10 mm measured along short axis, well defined margin, heterogenicity, absence of central hilar sign and a colour power doppler index grade of 2–3 are the predicting characteristics of a malignant lymph node as described by Shafiek et al. [4].

A systematic review and meta-analysis done by Agarwal et al. evaluating the diagnostic utility of endobronchial ultrasound features in differentiating malignant from benign lymph node found that presence of coagulation necrosis and absence of central hilar structure are the most important characteristic ultrasound features for diagnosing malignant lymph node [5].

Elastography is a new technology where stiffness of the tissue is used to assess the pathology of a lesion. This has opened new avenues to be used in EBUS to differentiate a benign lymph node from a malignant lymph node. They are of two types: (i) strain elastography imaging (ii) shear wave elastography imaging. Strain imaging is now available for endoscopic elastography. It is described as E-mode and they have different colour elastic coding for nodal characterization. Based on the nodal hardness they have been colour coded as blue, green and red for hard, intermediate and soft nodal tissues respectively. Elasto-sonography equipped with ultrasound devices will give better imaging and characteristics of the nature of lesions [6]. Elastographic patterns were evaluated by Izumo using a new endoscopic ultrasound processor. They evaluated 75 patients and found that the sensitivity, specificity, positive predictive value, negative predictive value, and diagnostic accuracy rates were 100%, 92.3%, 94.6%, 100%, and 96.7%, respectively, with the high negative predictive value potentially minimizing unnecessary punctures. Hence, they came to the conclusion that endobronchial ultrasound elastography of mediastinal and hilar lymph nodes are a form of non-invasive technology that can be useful in predicting nodal metastasis during EBUS-TBNA [7].

4.2 Artifacts in EBUS

It is essential to identify if any artifacts are present while performing EBUS-TBNA. Reverberation artifacts are commonly seen while performing EBUS when the contact between the airway wall and balloon of the bronchoscope probe is lost. They are usually seen as bright parallel lines occurring at regular intervals. Tadpole tail sign and acoustic shadow sign are some of the attenuation artifacts that are observed while performing EBUS and hence one should be aware of it. In tadpole sign the area below the low impedance structure like necrotic node appears as a linear bright line. Acoustic shadow is opposite of tadpole tail sign i.e., the area below the high impedance appears as dark shadow.

There are few significant and clinically relevant lines that occur during ultrasound and novice ultrasonologist must be aware of it. "A" lines are hyperechoic horizontal lines which are seen between ribs shadows and are equally spaced with a distance equal to skin-pleura width. These are reverberation artifacts observed while performing EBUS. "B" lines originate from the pleural surface and spread vertically to the edge of the screen without fading. These are also considered reverberation artifacts. "E" lines look similar to B-lines and are due to subcutaneous emphysema and hence originate below the skin surface.

References

1. Zhi X, Chen J, Xie F, Sun J, Herth FJF. Diagnostic value of endobronchial ultrasound image features: a specialized review. Endosc Ultrasound. 2021;10(1):3–18. https://doi.org/10.4103/eus.eus_43_20.

2. Ayub II, Mohan A, Madan K, Hadda V, Jain D, Khilnani GC, Guleria R. Identification of specific EBUS sonographic characteristics for predicting benign mediastinal lymph nodes. Clin Respir J. 2018;12(2):681–90. https://doi.org/10.1111/crj.12579. Epub 2016 Nov 15. PMID: 27805323.
3. Dhooria S, Agarwal R, Aggarwal AN, Bal A, Gupta N, Gupta D. Differentiating tuberculosis from sarcoidosis by sonographic characteristics of lymph nodes on endobronchial ultrasonography: a study of 165 patients. J Thorac Cardiovasc Surg. 2014;148(2):662–7. https://doi.org/10.1016/j.jtcvs.2014.01.028.
4. Shafiek H, Fiorentino F, Peralta AD, et al. Real-time prediction of mediastinal lymph node malignancy by endobronchial ultrasound. Arch Bronconeumol. 2014;50(6):228–34. https://doi.org/10.1016/j.arbres.2013.12.002.
5. Agrawal S, Goel AD, Gupta N, Lohiya A, Gonuguntla HK. Diagnostic utility of endobronchial ultrasound (EBUS) features in differentiating malignant and benign lymph nodes—a systematic review and meta-analysis. Respir Med. 2020;171:106097. https://doi.org/10.1016/j.rmed.2020.106097.
6. Jiang JH, Turner JF Jr, Huang JA. Endobronchial ultrasound elastography: a new method in endobronchial ultrasound-guided transbronchial needle aspiration. J Thorac Dis. 2015;7(Suppl 4):S272–8. https://doi.org/10.3978/j.issn.2072-1439.2015.12.53.
7. Izumo T, Sasada S, Chavez C, Matsumoto Y, Tsuchida T. Endobronchial ultrasound elastography in the diagnosis of mediastinal and hilar lymph nodes. Jpn J Clin Oncol. 2014;44(10):956–62. https://doi.org/10.1093/jjco/hyu105.

5 Transbronchial Needle Aspiration

Transbronchial needle aspiration (TBNA) is a bronchoscopy technique which is performed to obtain both histological or cytological sample specimen. Based on the type or site of aspiration required, needles of different sizes are passed either through the barrel of the rigid bronchoscope or through the working channel of the flexible bronchoscope. The tissues that can be obtained from various sites of lung through TBNA technique are like endobronchial tumours, lymph nodes, tissues adjacent to the airway wall and the peripheral lung nodules. The main purpose of transbronchial needle aspiration is to aid in the diagnosis and staging of bronchogenic carcinoma. Diagnosis of endobronchial tumours, submucosal lesions, externally compressing central airway tumours and the staging of mediastinal lymph nodes in bronchogenic carcinoma are all performed by transbronchial needle aspiration technique.

Staging of cancer especially, non-small cell lung cancer (NSCLC) is required for therapeutic options like chemotherapy, radiotherapy, and curative surgery. This calls for multiple station mediastinal lymph node sampling so as to determine the stage of lung cancer and to prepare decision tree regarding treatment or palliative therapy. Though contrast enhanced computed tomography (CECT) and positron emission tomography (PET) scans aids in determining the extent of anatomical involvement and metastatic progression, but still histopathological diagnosis is required

M. M. Mohapatra, P. Upadhya, *Handbook of Endobronchial Ultrasound*, https://doi.org/10.1007/978-981-96-0531-6_5

to confirm the type of lung cancer and for management by the newly available options of targeted and molecular chemotherapy.

Conventional TBNA is usually performed through flexible bronchoscope. This is performed under direct visualization of the airway lumen by the bronchoscope. The widening of the carina seen in flexible bronchoscope is an indication of enlarged subcarinal node. Therefore, conventional TBNA can sample and assess only subcarinal lymph node while other mediastinal nodes cannot be approached. A few intrapulmonary mass lesions which cause external compression can also be sampled by conventional TBNA under fluoroscopy guidance. Mondoni et al. in their systematic review and meta- analysis on yield of conventional TBNA in peripheral pulmonary lesions done by fluoroscopy guidance found that conventional TBNA is a safe and useful diagnostic technique for peripheral lung lesions and the accuracy is higher in cases where chest tomography showed CT bronchus sign or pulmonary lesions with diameter >3 cm [1]. The needles that are used for conventional TBNA are also different from that used for EBUS- TBNA.

Mediastinoscopy is considered as a gold standard diagnostic procedure for mediastinal lymph nodes, but this needs general anaesthesia. Hence, restaging of the nodes after induction chemotherapy and radiotherapy may be challenging to perform using mediastinoscopy owing to its risk involved. EBUS TBNA has an advantage over other techniques as it can be performed under minimal sedation and there is no harmful effect on repeating the procedure for restaging. A meta-analysis on diagnostic yield of conventional TBNA in NSCLC for mediastinal node was found to be between 14% and 100% [1, 2]. The technique of TBNA performed by EBUS versus conventional method was compared to assess the diagnostic yield. Zhu T et al. in their meta-analysis found that EBUS TBNA performed better than conventional TBNA with shorter duration of aspiration time and had higher sensitivity with OR = 2.72, 95% CI:1.72–4.30 [3]. However, a meta-analysis by Yan JH suggested that there is no significant difference in the diagnostic yield between both the TBNA technique and the pooled sensitivity was 0.90 (95% CI 0.85–0.94) and 0.76 (95% CI 0.68–0.82), pooled specificity was 0.75 (95% CI

0.60–0.87) and 0.94 (95% CI 0.86–0.98),diagnostic odds ratio (DOR) was 75.38 (95% CI 16.38–346.97) and 108.17 (95% CI 13.84–845.35), and area under curve (AUC) was 0.9339 and 0.9732 for EBUS-TBNA group and conventional TBNA group, respectively [4].

Malignant lesions which are visible on bronchoscopy in endobronchial lumen can be exophytic, submucosal in nature or present as extrinsic compression. Endobronchial biopsy, bronchial brushing and bronchoalveolar lavage are carried out for diagnosis of these lesions. However, studies have shown that the yield of TBNA in endobronchial tumours range from 69% to 96%. The yield of endobronchial biopsy increases from 90% to 95% on using conventional biopsy with TBNA in exophytic lesions. In cases of submucosal lesions and extrinsic compression the yield increased from 30–70% to 85–95% when both bronchial brushing and TBNA were used together [5, 6].

Extrinsic compression of the airway which occur due to peripheral tumors can be diagnosed by conventional methods like bronchial brushing and bronchoalveolar lavage. Tumors, which have infiltrated the airway walls can yield better results with bronchial brushing. A study by Acharya K V et al. showed that bronchial brushing had a positive predictive value of 61.29% and diagnostic accuracy of 55.74% in lung cancer as compared to biopsy and bronchial washing. Bronchial brushing showed better yield for both central and peripheral tumors and tumours showing mucosal wall irregularity and infiltration [7]. Endobronchial biopsy or fine needle aspiration biopsy (FNAB) can be performed for tumors that have exfoliated to the airway lumen as endobronchial polypoid growth. Pulmonary salivary gland type tumors and carcinoid tumors are though considered as uncommon variant of lung cancer, but these tumors occur centrally with endobronchial involvement [8]. Hence, they are better diagnosed by fine needle aspiration biopsy and can be managed by surgical resection. Conventional transbronchial needle aspiration can be used to sample those tumors which do not infiltrate the airway mucosa, but due to external compression bronchial brushing is not possible. Needle aspiration beyond the point of compression can be performed either by TBNA or by fluoroscopy guidance. Studies examining the yield of these types of tumors which can be approached by radial EBUS, and it was reported by Ali MS et al. that the diagnostic yield is as high as 70.6% [9].

Small cell lung cancer is staged differently from NSCLC. It is classified as limited stage (limited to a single radiation port) or extensive stage (extending beyond a single radiation field). In small cell lung cancer, TBNA of mediastinal lymph nodes is performed for primary diagnosis rather than for mediastinal staging. Besides the role of TBNA in diagnosing and staging of lung cancer, malignant lymphadenopathy is also evaluated for lymphoma. It has also been used in diagnosing benign lesions. The most common benign adenopathy which were diagnosed by TBNA include sarcoidosis and mycobacterium tuberculosis.

5.1 EBUS Needles (Fig. 5.1)

The needles that are used to perform TBNA are of various gauges. A long needle is preferred in lesions present in the central airways to have better penetration through the airway and into the lymph node or mass. A shorter needle is preferred for peripheral nodules due to the risk of pneumothorax. The transbronchial needle consist of a bevelled needle which can be fully retracted into a plastic protective sheath. A Luer lock system is present at the end of the needle to prevent from being accidentally deployed or retracted and to apply negative suction during needle aspiration procedure to retrieve the sample material. The TBNA needles are usually passed through the working channel of a flexible bronchoscope or the barrel of a rigid bronchoscope. It is essential to check the proper functioning of the needles before deploying them to the working channel. Hence, endoscopy assistant or technician must check whether the needle is broken, bent or stuck with residual material from prior procedures before passing it through the bronchoscope if it is a reusable needle.

The EBUS TBNA needles are not reusable but in low-income countries where there is substantial financial burden without availability of insurance facility, reuse of EBUS TBNA needle will reduce the cost incurred. This is an essential step before each

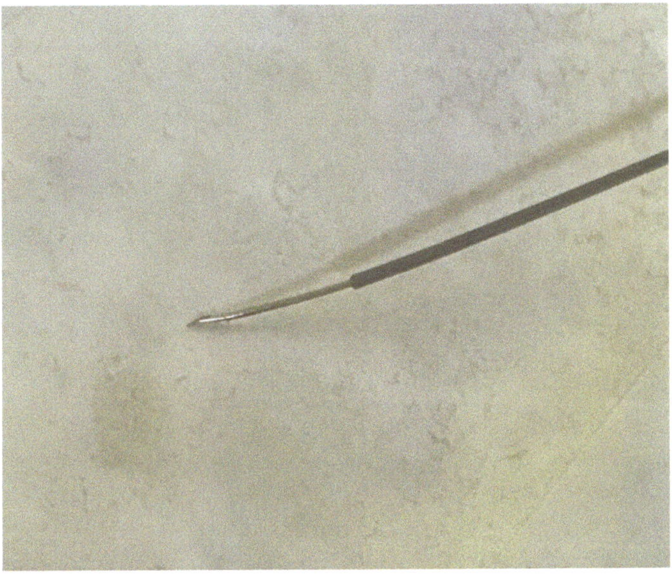

Fig. 5.1 The endobronchial ultrasound linear probe needle with bevelled end

use as the needle may fail to open once inside the airways or the yield of the aspiration material may be inadequate and unsatisfactory. A damaged or malfunctioned needle may cause the needle to pass through a different route causing damage to the working channel. It is therefore recommended to flush the needle thoroughly following each use to reduce the presence of any residue from the prior procedure so that a good quality specimen can be obtained. Also, it is important to ensure that the bronchoscope is in neutral position whenever the needle is passed through the working channel to avoid damage to the channel.

Various needles sizes are used for EBUS TBNA ranging from 19G to 25G. There are 19G, 21G, 22G and 25G needles available for use for EBUS TBNA. According to American College of Chest Physician guidelines 2016 for use of EBUS needle, it was recommended to use either 21G or 22G. However, the yield of the sample was found to be more with 21G needle compared to 22G according to various studies. It is also seen that the use of the size of the needle may vary based on the type of lesion. It was observed that the yield of sample was good when 19G needle is used for cases like sarcoidosis or lymphoma but the sample may be bloody [10].

5.2 EBUS TBNA in Benign Adenopathy

Sarcoidosis: Adenopathy is most commonly seen in stage I and stage II sarcoidosis with stage I having only adenopathy while stage II having adenopathy with interstitial changes. Traditionally, sarcoidosis can be diagnosed based on clinical presentation, radiographic abnormalities, and supportive ancillary testing. With the advent of bronchoscopy, transbronchial cryobiospies, endobronchial biopsies, bronchoalveolar lavage and TBNA have become the mainstay to diagnose pulmonary sarcoidosis. Literature search shows that the diagnostic yield is higher with TBNA in stage I sarcoidosis while transbronchial and endobronchial biopsies yield are higher in stage II sarcoidosis. In stage II sarcoidosis, TBNA has only additive role. The diagnostic yield of EBUS TBNA ranged from 54% to 93% as suggested by Agarwal R et al. in a meta-analysis on sarcoidosis [11].

Tuberculosis: Mediastinal lymphadenopathy may be a presenting feature in mycobacterium tuberculosis and nontuberculous mycobacterium tuberculosis in reference to HIV patients. A bronchoscopy diagnosis particularly EBUS TBNA is done in case of patients who are sputum smear negative for acid fast bacilli (AFB). It was observed in a study that patients who were HIV-1 positive with lymphadenopathy and were sputum smear negative, the diagnosis of tuberculosis was made in 87% in combination with smear, histology and culture by using conventional bronchoscopy TBNA [11]. In non-HIV patients with sputum smear negative for AFB, the yield of TBNA was around 80% in a tuberculosis endemic country [11, 12]. A multi-centric study done by Navani N et al. on utility of EBUS TBNA for diagnosing tuberculous intrathoracic lymphadenitis found that diagnosis of tuberculosis could be demonstrated in 146 patients out of 156 patients with cytological specimens (94%; 95% CI 88–97%) [13].

Lymphoma: Mediastinal and hilar lymph nodes are involved in 85% of all cases of Hodgkin's lymphoma and 45% of all cases of

Non-Hodgkin's lymphoma. EBUS TBNA is an important tool for diagnosing and subtyping of mediastinal lymphoma. The majority of lymphoma cases manifest as generalized lymph node enlargement allowing for surgical biopsy of peripheral lymph nodes under local anaesthesia. However, isolated enlargement of mediastinal lymph nodes is a rare presentation in some patients. The diagnostic yield of EBUS-TBNA for mediastinal lymphoma in several single centered studies ranged from 48% to 98%. Dhooria et al. in a retrospective multi centric study found that the sensitivity for detection of lymphoma by EBUS TBNA was around 73% which was lower and similar to other studies [14].

5.3 Insertion of Conventional TBNA Needle Technique

There are four most common technique for needle insertion while performing TBNA. These needle insertion techniques are mainly performed by flexible bronchoscopy with conventional TBNA. These techniques are as follows:

(a) Hub method: This is the most common method applied by many clinicians. In this method, the hub of the needle catheter is brought close to the airway wall so that the catheter is perpendicular to the airway wall and does not cause mucosal injury. The bronchoscope is then made to be in position and the needle is advanced through the airway wall to reach the target. The needle is passed several times through the target with subsequent application of suction. The TBNA needle along with the catheter is then removed from the airway and the bronchoscope.
(b) Jabbing method: After the needle is introduced through the working channel and the catheter hub becomes visualized in the airways, the needle is then advanced such that the bevel end is clearly seen. The catheter and the actual needle are then retracted to the working channel of the bronchoscope with only the bevelled portion of the needle is visible in the airway protruding from the sheath. The entire apparatus (needle, catheter, and the bronchoscope) is then advanced forward en

bloc to the site of interest. The entire length of the needle is then pushed forward to penetrate the airway wall. The needle is then jabbed and a Luer lock syringe is used to apply suction on the needle to retrieve the aspirated material.

(c) Piggy back method: This technique requires that the bronchoscope is positioned in proximity of the site of interest. The catheter is then advanced till the hub is visible and then the needle is ejected and locked at the desired place. The entire bronchoscope with needle is placed perpendicular to the airway wall and advanced so that the needle penetrates the mucosa. It is essential to ensure that the needle does not migrate proximally or distally while advancing the bronchoscope. It is also important to minimize the length of the catheter and needle beyond the distal end of the bronchoscope as it becomes difficult to manipulate into the desired position to optimize the yield and minimize airway trauma.

(d) Cough method: In this technique the patient is allowed to cough to facilitate the penetration of the needle into the airway wall. This cough guided method can be combined with other methods to get a better yield. It is also recommended to attempt 3–5 needle aspiration rates of each target for optimizing the yield of the sample specimen.

5.3.1 EBUS TBNA Technique

This is a real time technique where simultaneous ultrasonographic images are visualized and sampling material are obtained from the lesion. The EBUS bronchoscope transducer can detect only five out of seven layers of the main airway wall structure [3]. The tip of the bronchoscope which consists of the transducer and remains in direct contact with the balloon can be flexed sideways, up, or down with the help of flexion lever.

The ultrasonic images are adjusted accordingly using the scroll knob on the keyboard. As the EBUS bronchoscope is grazed against the airway wall from distal to proximal airways, various anatomical structures are visible. Thus, from the distal left main bronchus the left pulmonary artery is seen at 10 O'clock position, aorta at the 7 O'clock position while the left atrium is seen between 1 and 3

O'clock position. When the EBUS scope is pulled further proximally the esophagus is seen at 6 O'clock position while near the bifurcation the main pulmonary artery and its branches can be visualized ventrally. Therefore, the descending aorta, oesophagus and the vertebral column appear behind the proximal left bronchus when the tip of bronchoscope is placed dorsally. On the right side, as the probe of the EBUS reaches the origin of the upper lobe bronchus from bronchus intermedius, ventrally the right pulmonary artery and vein crosses from right to left accompanied by ascending aorta to the left and superior venacava to the right. At the right tracheobronchial angle, the azygos vein is located dorsally to the right of esophagus. The radial EBUS probe however is helpful in identifying any parenchymal lesions around the bronchus.

The curved transducer of EBUS TBNA bronchoscope usually obtain images at 65° angle which extends from proximal to distal. An indicator in the ultrasound image screen present in the extreme right top of the screen marks the instrument channel opening of the endoscope. This is the position for entry of the TBNA needles. A disposable inflatable balloon attached to the transducer is filled with sterile saline water to improve the clarity of ultrasound images by acoustic coupling between mucosal wall and ultrasound probe (Fig. 5.2).

The needles have multiple dimpling to enhance echogenicity and improve visualization on the screen. Once the EBUS bron-

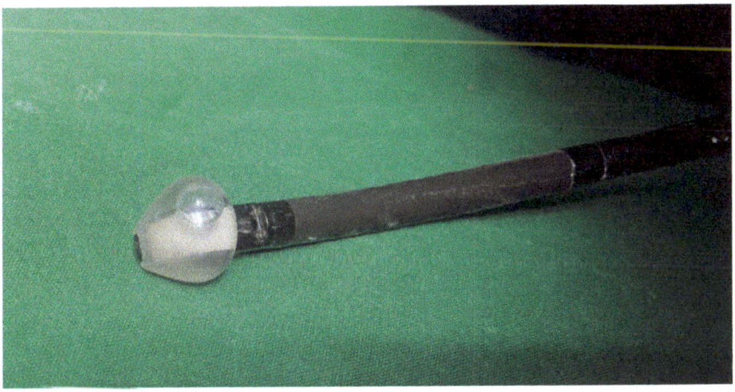

Fig. 5.2 The inflatable balloon attached to the transducer of convex probe filled with saline

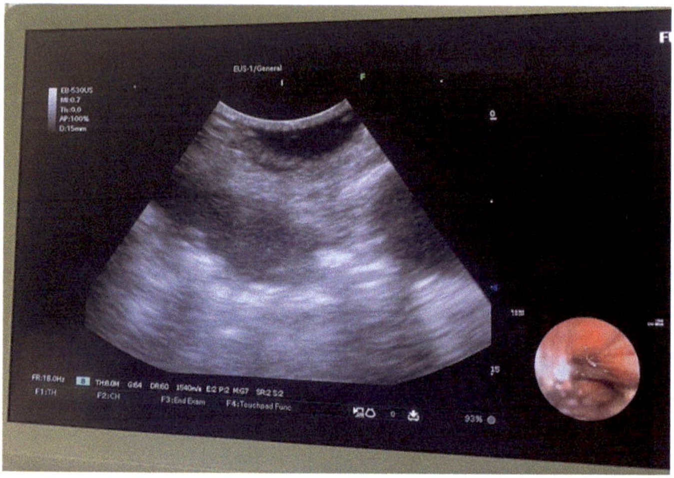

Fig. 5.3 The ultrasound image of linear probe with deflated balloon when adherent to airway wall

choscope enters the trachea, the bronchoscope is flexed to the target area so that the transducer can get adequate contact with the airway wall. The fluid filled balloon on the transducer becomes visible on the ultrasound images as curved shadow (Fig. 5.3).

The bronchoscope is then rotated and grazed in the airway wall to obtain the images of the targeted lymph node. The balloon is then inflated to obtain good contact between airway wall and probe. It is important to note that the optimum volume of saline required should be such that it enables circumferential contact of balloon with the bronchial wall. Over inflation of the balloon will cause bronchial wall structures to compress or the balloon may burst.

Colour doppler is used to differentiate blood vessels from lymph node. The diameter of the lymph node is then measured by freezing the images. The bronchoscope is kept in neutral position and the needle is passed through the working channel. The needle is then secured by moving the connecting slider to the opposite side until you hear a clicking sound (Fig. 5.4).

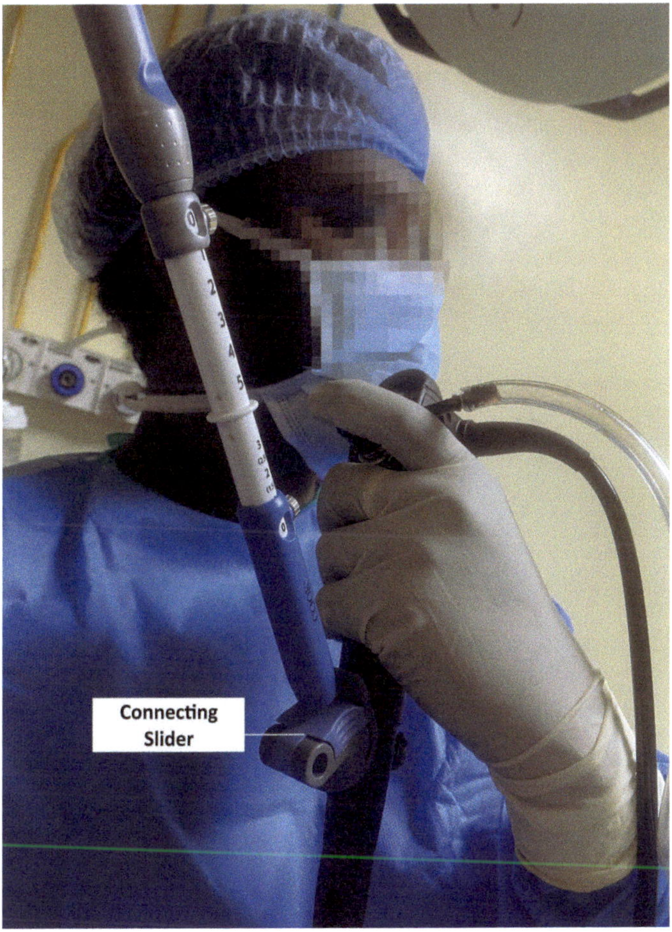

Fig. 5.4 The connecting slider connecting the EBUS needle with the bronchoscope

The length of the sheath is then adjusted using the needle sheath adjuster. The needle sheath adjuster slider is moved down to the desired position so that the tip of the sheath is just visible in the white light. The length of the needle to be advanced then can be adjusted accordingly from the ultrasound images. Usually,

2 cm to 4 cm is the desired length for the needle to be adjusted for adequate penetration. The needle is then advanced till the ultrasound images disappear and then both the scope and the needle are advanced together till the ultrasound images reappear (Fig. 5.5).

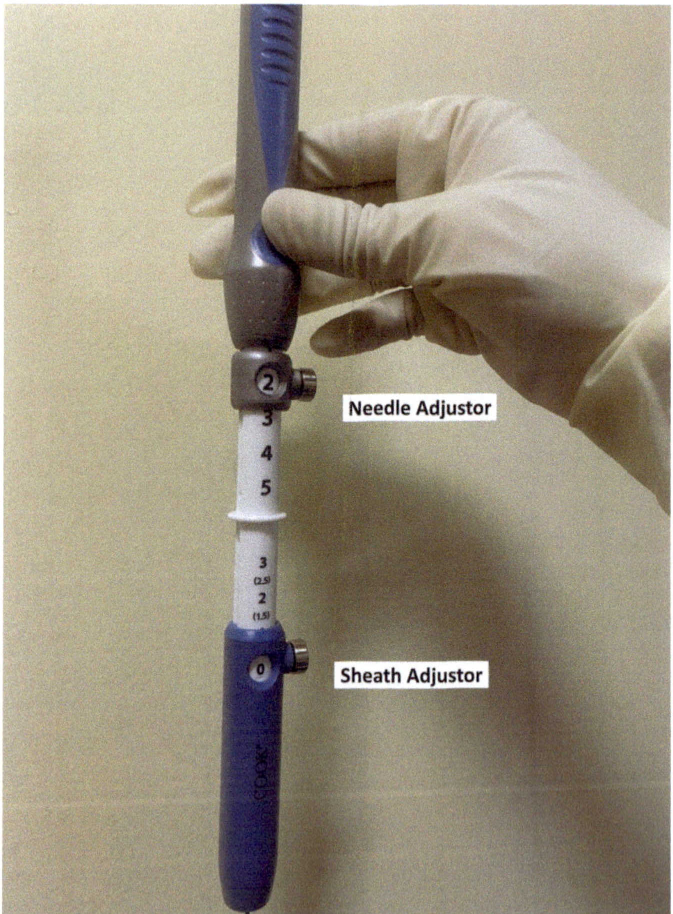

Fig. 5.5 The sheath adjuster knob and the needle adjuster knob

The needle is then advanced further into the lymph node. The stylet is pulled out and the suction syringe is then attached to apply suction. The needle is ready to be jabbed to start sampling for the lymph node. The suction is removed and the above procedure is followed in a reverse order.

5.3.2 Factors Affecting TBNA Yield

The yields of TBNA vary widely based on difference in patient population, clinical experience, and technical expertise. The higher the disease prevalence in a patient population, higher is the yield of TBNA. The greater yield is also seen if the node is at an accessible position and of bigger size. Generally, the right paratracheal node and the subcarinal lymph node are the ones which are quite accessible and are thought to have a higher yield of specimen sample. A lymph node size of about 2 cm or above also gives a better yield if the physician is a beginner. However, in malignancy lymph node of size >5 mm in short axis can be sampled by EBUS. There are also technical factors that determines the positivity of a sample specimen. They include the quality and use of image guidance, needle size, number of passes used for obtaining a good sample, sample preparation and presence of an experienced cytopathologist during the on-site procedure.

A greater diagnostic yield occurs when peripheral TBNA is done by fluoroscopic guidance. EBUS TBNA has a better yield for mediastinal, paratracheal and pretracheal lymph nodes compared to blind bronchoscopic TBNA. Staging of mediastinal nodes when assisted with PET scanning improves sensitivity, specificity, and diagnostic accuracy as per studies. The transbronchial needles are mainly used to obtain both histological and cytological specimens. Histological core needles varies from size of 18–19 gauge while cytological needles varies from 20–22 gauge. Studies have shown that the diagnostic yield are better with use of cytological needles rather than histological needles. A 19-gauge needle can be used for better sampling of distance nodes also [15, 16].

References

1. Mondoni M, Sotgiu G, Bonifazi M, et al. Transbronchial needle aspiration in peripheral pulmonary lesions: a systematic review and meta-analysis. Eur Respir J. 2016;48(1):196–204. https://doi.org/10.1183/13993003.00051-2016.
2. Detterbeck F, Jantz M, Wallace M, et al. Invasive mediastinal staging of lung cancer: ACCP evidence-based clinical practice guidelines (2nd edition). Chest. 2007;132:202S–20S.
3. Holty J-E, Kuschner W, Gould M. Accuracy of transbronchial needle aspiration for mediastinal staging of non-small cell lung cancer: a meta-analysis. Thorax. 2005;60:949–55.
4. Zhu T, Zhang X, Xu J, et al. Endobronchial ultrasound guided-transbronchial needle aspiration vs. conventional transbronchial needle aspiration in the diagnosis of mediastinal masses: a meta-analysis. Mol Clin Oncol. 2014;2(1):151–5. https://doi.org/10.3892/mco.2013.206.
5. Yan JH, Pan L, Chen XL, et al. Endobronchial ultrasound versus conventional transbronchial needle aspiration in the diagnosis of mediastinal lymphadenopathy: a meta-analysis. Springerplus. 2016;5(1):1716. https://doi.org/10.1186/s40064-016-3348-1. Published 2016 Oct 5.
6. Dasgupta A, Jain P, Minai O, et al. Utility of transbronchial needle aspiration in the diagnosis of endobronchial lesions. Chest. 1999;115:1237–41.
7. Gullon J, Fernandez R, Medina A, et al. Transbronchial needle aspiration in bronchogenic carcinoma with visible lesions: diagnostic yield and cost. Arch Bronconeumol. 2003;39:496–500.
8. Acharya KV, Unnikrishnan B, Shenoy A, Holla R. Utility of various bronchoscopic modalities in lung cancer diagnosis. Asian Pac J Cancer Prev. 2017;18(7):1931–6. https://doi.org/10.22034/APJCP.2017.18.7.1931. Published 2017 Jul 27.
9. Wahidi MM, Herth F, Yasufuku K, et al. Technical aspects of endobronchial ultrasound-guided transbronchial needle aspiration: CHEST guideline and expert panel report. Chest. 2016;149(3):816–35. https://doi.org/10.1378/chest.15-1216.
10. Aldera AP, Schubert PT. Endobronchial masses encountered on fine-needle aspiration biopsy: a focus on unusual entities. Diagn Cytopathol. 2020;48(8):807–12. https://doi.org/10.1002/dc.24437.
11. Ali MS, Trick W, Mba BI, Mohananey D, Sethi J, Musani AI. Radial endobronchial ultrasound for the diagnosis of peripheral pulmonary lesions: a systematic review and meta-analysis. Respirology. 2017;22(3):443–53. https://doi.org/10.1111/resp.12980.
12. Agarwal R, Srinivasan A, Aggarwal AN, Gupta D. Efficacy and safety of convex probe EBUS-TBNA in sarcoidosis: a systematic review and meta-analysis. Respir Med. 2012;106(6):883–92. https://doi.org/10.1016/j.rmed.2012.02.014.

13. Harkin T, Ciotoli C, Addrizzo-Harris D, et al. Transbronchial needle aspiration (TBNA) in patients infected with HIV. Am J Respir Crit Care Med. 1998;157:1913–8.
14. Bilacerolu S, Gunel O, Eri N, et al. Transbronchial needle aspiration in diagnosing intrathoracic tuberculous lymphadenitis. Chest. 2004;126:259–67.
15. Centinkaya E, Yildiz P, Kadakal F, et al. Transbronchial needle aspiration in the diagnosis of intrathoracic lymphadenopathy. Respiration. 2002;69:335–3.
16. Hermens FH, Van Engelenburg TC, Visser FJ, Thunnissen FB, Termeer R, Janssen JP. Diagnostic yield of transbronchial histology needle aspiration in patients with mediastinal lymph node enlargement. Respiration. 2003;70(6):631–5. https://doi.org/10.1159/000075210.

Linear EBUS

6

EBUS bronchoscope is difficult to manipulate in the airways owing to its thickness, limited flexibility and the forward oblique view angulation. The flexibility is further compromised if a needle set is introduced into the working channel of the bronchoscope. Also, it is difficult for the EBUS scope to enter into right and left upper lobes as well as right middle lobe. The balloon present in the EBUS bronchoscope is inflated with normal saline to help in obtaining good ultrasound images when in contact with the bronchial wall.

6.1 Linear EBUS Procedure Proper

The execution of an EBUS procedure can differ across various settings influenced by the accessibility of resources and expertise of the interventionist. After an overnight period of fast, patient is received in the bronchoscopy suite and nebulized with 2.5 ml of salbutamol nebulization. Patient is then given topical lignocaine (10%) spray in the oropharynx after a gap of 15 min following nebulization. Patient is made to lie down in supine position on the operating table.

An intravenous line is secured and arrangements are made to monitor vitals like blood pressure, oxygen saturation and electrocardiogram. The oral suction system is kept ready before starting the procedure. The bronchoscopist stands at the head end of the patient.

M. M. Mohapatra, P. Upadhya, *Handbook of Endobronchial Ultrasound*, https://doi.org/10.1007/978-981-96-0531-6_6

Oxygen delivery system is attached to the patient and the bronchoscope is cleaned and kept ready to be used by the technician or the trained nurse. Patient is then administered drugs like intravenous midazolam dexmedetomidine and fentanyl for conscious sedation.

EBUS bronchoscope is then introduced through oral route after fixing mouth gag. 2 ml of 1% lignocaine is pushed through the bronchoscope while the bronchoscope passes through the vocal cord and main airways. A quick inspection of the airways is done and then bronchoscope is grazed on the trachea and the medial bronchial walls with the ultrasound probe facing the walls after crossing the vocal cords up to the division on both side of the main bronchus. The probe is grazed on the tracheal wall till the origin of the left side main bronchus to look for left upper paratracheal and left lower paratracheal nodes (Fig. 6.1).

The scope is than rotated to the right with the convex probe grazing the medial wall till the origin of the right main bronchus to identify the 4R nodes (Fig. 6.2).

The subcarinal nodes are then visualized using EBUS and the vascular structures with colour Doppler to avoid puncture of vital vascular structures (Fig. 6.3).

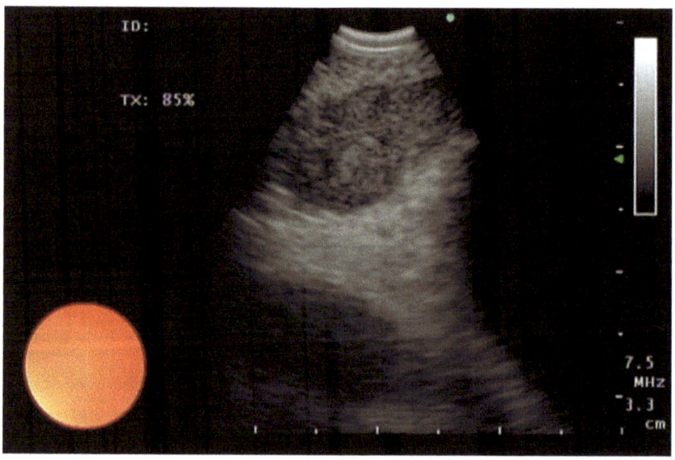

Fig. 6.1 Image of left lower paratracheal node as visualized by ultrasound in linear EBUS. (Photo Courtesy- Dr. Harshith R Rao)

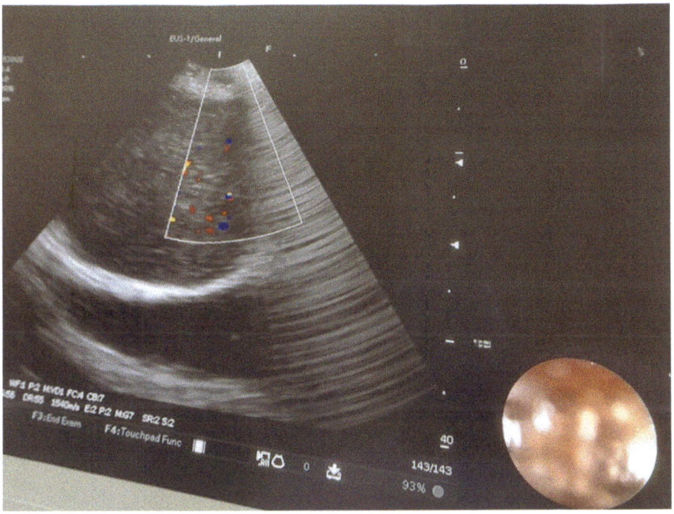

Fig. 6.2 Image of right lower paratracheal node as visualized by EBUS

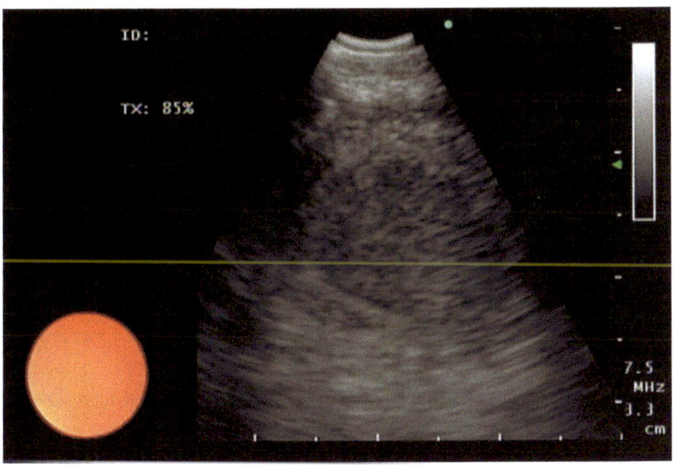

Fig. 6.3 Image of subcarinal node as visualized by EBUS. (Photo Courtesy-Dr. Harshith R Rao)

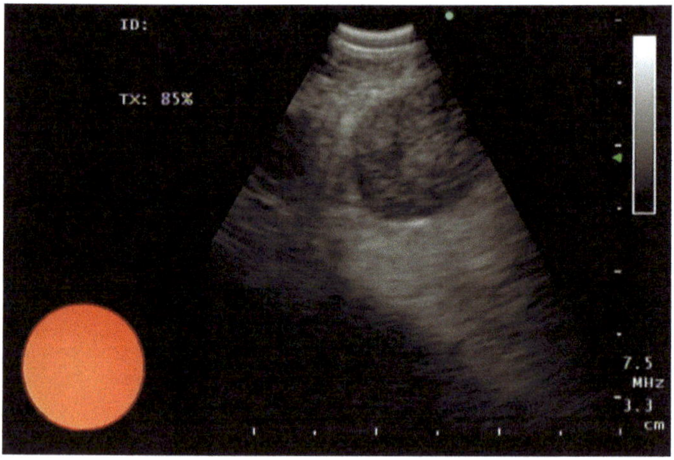

Fig. 6.4 Image of hilar node as visualized by EBUS. (Photo Courtesy- Dr. Harshith R Rao)

The probe is the further grazed down on both right and left main bronchus to locate the hilar nodes (Fig. 6.4).

The size, shape and characteristics of the lymph node is then noted. The needle along with the sheath is first secured and under real time ultrasound guidance the needle is introduced into the node. Sometimes the bronchial cartilage may interfere during needle penetration which is taken care of by the internal stylet present in the needle. The needle depth should be measured accurately before inserting the needle to prevent puncture of vascular structure.

The needle is moved back and forth in the target lesion about 10–15 times on each pass with a minimum of 10 agitation. Around three to four passes are required for each target node to get an adequate sample for diagnosis and molecular study. The needle is then fully retracted into the needle sheath and finally the needle set is removed from the working channel. A 20 ml vacuum syringe is provided with EBUS and negative pressure is applied through this vacuum suction syringe to obtain material from TBNA.

6.2 Rapid On-site Evaluation (ROSE) and Sampling

The type of sampling depends on the purpose of procedure. The sample aspirated from node/lesion is expressed on a glass slide by pushing air through a 10 ml syringe and smears are prepared. Half of the slides are then dried and the other half are fixed with alcohol (95% ethanol). After the first pass/attempt rapid on-site evaluation is performed on one of the alcohol fixed slide smear. With the help of rapid stain which needs smearing of the glass slide with cytological sample uses one of the stain (Diff-Quick, toluidine blue, Giemsa stain and other stains). The smear is then visualized under the microscope. The ROSE smear can be interpreted by a cytotechnologist/pathologist who can help to determine the adequacy and representativeness of the material for interpretation. A second or even a third pass/attempt can be made if the material is inadequate/non representative. The other advantage of ROSE is that it gives provisional idea about the nature of pathology: Thus during the second pass/attempt extra material can be collected for ancillary tests (Cell block (Formalin)/Flow cytometry (EDTA tube with PBS buffer)/(Molecular testing-normal saline). Samples for microbiological testing and culture are sent in normal saline and histopathological sample either in formalin or normal saline based on pathology. This procedure not only reduces sample loss but also improves accuracy and prevents the pain of repeating the procedure for patients to arrive at a diagnosis (Fig. 6.5).

The sampling of nodes needs a disease specific procedure which is mentioned as follows:

(i) Sampling for staging of lung cancer: The highest nodal station is sampled first in staging of lung cancer. Each node aspirate is prepared in separate slide and labelled. After each sampling the needle is flushed with normal saline to prevent false positivity due to prior sampling.
(ii) Lymphoma: The sampling of node needs three to four passes for each node. The sample is collected for flow cytometry which enables for establishing lymphocyte monoclonality.

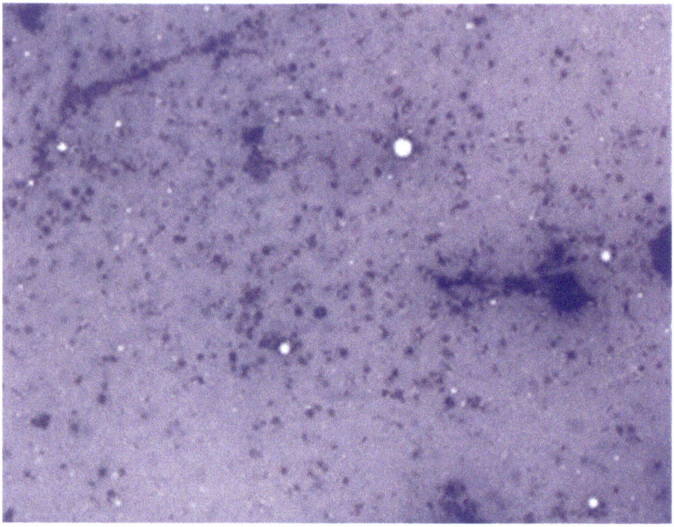

Fig. 6.5 Toluidine blue stained smear from a lymph node aspirate shows scattered lymphoid numerous cells during ROSE. From this smear one can opine that the material is representative and adequate if the FNAC target was a mediastinal node. (Photo Courtesy: Dr. Debasis Gocchait)

Samples are also collected and prepared for cell block in 10% buffered formalin.

(iii) Granulomatous diseases: Many granulomatous diseases present with hilar lymphadenopathy and more common being tuberculosis and sarcoidosis. In case of tuberculosis, 3–4 passes from each node is required by EBUS TBNA while in sarcoidosis three passes from two node and two passes from three nodes are required. Cell blocks are also prepared in case there is discrepancy in reports.

EUS-B-FNA: EBUS bronchoscope can be introduced into the esophagus to obtain sample from mediastinal lymph nodes in certain conditions where EBUS cannot be performed and is called endoscopic ultrasound with echobronchoscope guided FNA i.e.

"EUS -B-FNA". The lymph nodes that can be assessed by EUS-B-FNA are 4L,7,8,9 stations. The combination of EBUS-TBNA and EUS-B-FNA is otherwise called medical mediastinoscopy [1].

Transcutaneous mediastinal ultrasound was used 20 years back to obtain mediastinal lymph node sample mainly from prevascular, supra-aortal, and aorto-pulmonary window through a supra sternal approach. However due to its controversial use it is not done in most centers [2].

References

1. Dietrich CF, Annema JT, Clementsen P, Cui XW, Borst MM, Jenssen C. Ultrasound techniques in the evaluation of the mediastinum, part I: endoscopic ultrasound (EUS), endobronchial ultrasound (EBUS) and transcutaneous mediastinal ultrasound (TMUS), introduction into ultrasound techniques. J Thorac Dis. 2015;7(9):E311–25. https://doi.org/10.3978/j.issn.2072-1439.2015.09.40.
2. Hirche TO, Wagner TO, Dietrich CF. Mediastinal ultrasound: technique and possible applications. Med Klin (Munich). 2002;97:472–9.

Radial EBUS TBNA

7

EBUS with radial scanning miniature probe are nowadays used frequently owing to its minimal complications. The smaller diameter and high resolution of image allows it to be used for various indications. Some of the endobronchial tumors which are invisible on radiology can be detected and their extent as well as size, relationship with their surrounding structures can be well delineated by EBUS. This is helpful for patients who are at risk or have sputum cytology positive without radiological features. In situ lung cancer which are limited to the mucosa and not transgressing the lamina propria, as well as early lung cancer confined to the inner layers of the bronchial wall without infiltration to the cartilage can be detected by autofluorescence and narrow band imaging bronchoscopy procedures. It can also be detected with better precision by radial EBUS where alterations in the texture of the bronchial wall can be detected by using a 20 MHz radial probe (Fig. 7.1).

The disadvantage of autofluorescence in detecting positive results for benign lesions, scars, granulomas, and inflammation can be challenged with radial EBUS. Some of the macroscopically intact mucosa but submucosal and intramural tumor spread can be detected by EBUS. Hence, tumors that do not show any signs of infiltration to deep layers or involvement of lymph node can be considered as early malignancy and can be treated successfully using photodynamic therapy, endoluminal high dose radio-

M. M. Mohapatra, P. Upadhya, *Handbook of Endobronchial Ultrasound*, https://doi.org/10.1007/978-981-96-0531-6_7

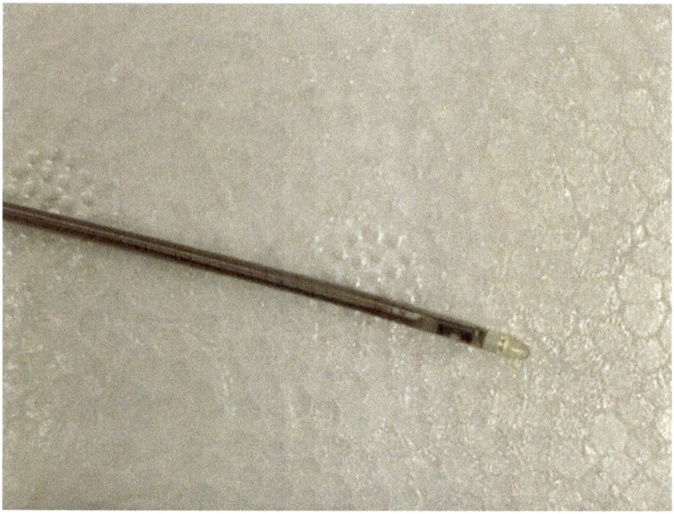

Fig. 7.1 Image of radial endobronchial ultrasound probe. (Photo Courtesy: Dr. Harshith R Rao)

therapy, brachytherapy or argon plasma coagulation. Studies have shown that tumors limited within the bronchial walls and staged by EBUS had complete remission on therapy and in long term follow-up.

EBUS is also found to be useful in locally advanced lung cancer. Patients with complete obstruction of the airway, EBUS helps to localize the base, extent of spread of the tumor and patency of the airway beyond stenosis. In regard to surgical planning, it is imperative to know the exact extent so that a decision regarding operability or palliative management can be taken. The combined use of auto fluorescence and EBUS has been found to be useful in determining the extent of spread. The involvement of the pulmonary vessels can also be detected by radial probe. The extent of infiltration of the vessel wall and pulsations of the wall as well as fluid inside can be detected by radial probe.

The infiltration of mediastinal structures by the tumor cells can be diagnosed by radial EBUS. Major mediastinal vessels infiltrations with tumors like aorta, vena cava, main pulmonary artery and vein which cannot be identified by radiographic method are better imaged with radial EBUS. This is an essential part of staging since decision for surgical procedures will be based on the involvement of mediastinal structures by the tumor spread.

7.1 Decision Plan for Use of Radial EBUS

Before proceeding towards performing radial EBUS, it is imperative to prepare a decision plan as to which patient will benefit from the procedure with minimal complications. Hence, CT scan thorax with axial, coronal and sagittal view of patients are reviewed before the procedure is planned. Patients who have peripherally located lesions, it is advisable to perform percutaneous needle aspiration. Though the chance of pneumothorax may be present but the yield of sample is likely to be promising. Patients with underlying lung disease like emphysema with peripheral lesion or centrally placed lesions, it is suitable to perform radial EBUS. Moreover, the experience and exposure of a bronchoscopist matters in taking a decision to perform radial EBUS.

Radial EBUS can be performed with or without using guide sheath. Institutions where there is availability of slim bronchoscope with a diameter of 4.2 mm, there is no need for guide sheath as the bronchoscope can be negotiated to subsegmental bronchus to performed the cytology and biopsy procedure for obtaining sample specimens. Radial EBUS can be performed with guide sheath in the presence or absence of fluoroscopy depending on the availability of the system.

7.2 Guide Sheath Preparation

The guide sheath kit consists of (1) a plastic tube with a metallic ring at one end called guide sheath (2) biopsy forceps (3) cytology brush (4) ET stopper and (5) ultrasound stopper. The ET stopper is used for biopsy forceps and cytology brush while the ultrasound stopper is used for radial ultrasound probe. The guide sheath is passed through the ET stopper and the stopper is made to slide till it reaches the proximal end of the guide sheath. Another ET stopper is made to pass over the cytology brush and fixed at a point so that the distal tip of the guide sheath coincides with the distal tip of the sheath covering the brush. In case of biopsy forceps, the ET stopper is fixed at a point where the distal end of the forceps can be opened. The ultrasound stopper is made to slide over the radial EBUS probe. The probe is then passed through the guide sheath and the ultrasound stopper is fixed at a point at which the distal end of the probe comes out of the sheath (Fig. 7.2).

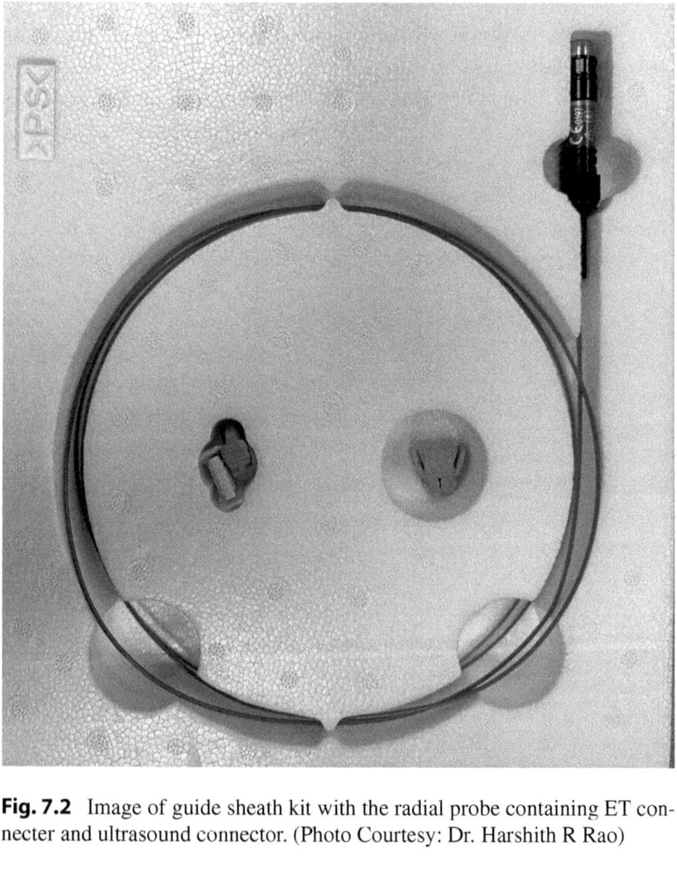

Fig. 7.2 Image of guide sheath kit with the radial probe containing ET connecter and ultrasound connector. (Photo Courtesy: Dr. Harshith R Rao)

7.3 Radial EBUS Procedure Proper

Radial EBUS procedure is usually performed in operation theatre or in bronchoscopy suite with the help of anaesthesiologist. This procedure is performed under moderate sedation through endotracheal tube or laryngeal mask depending on the competency of bronchoscopist and presence of anaesthesia support. Peripheral radial EBUS can be performed in various ways based on the location of the nodule and experience of the bronchoscopist. Once the radial EBUS probe is introduced into the lesion, the ultrasound console shows a rounded lesion with snow storm appearance (Fig. 7.3).

After introducing the bronchoscope, the guide sheath along with the radial EBUS probe is passed through the working channel. Once the bronchoscope reaches the segmental bronchus, the guide sheath along with the radial EBUS probe are pushed further to look for any luminal or extraluminal pathology. At times where there is a need to change the direction of the probe, a double hinged directional curette is introduced into the working channel with the guide sheath. The guide sheath is then left at the desired

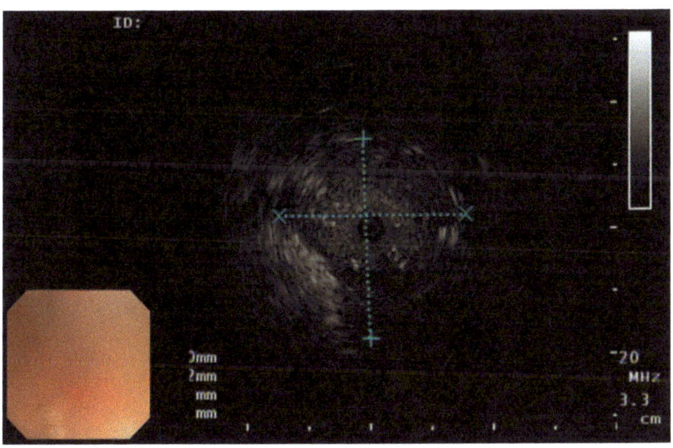

Fig. 7.3 Ultrasound image of the peripheral lung lesion as seen by radial EBUS. (Photo Courtesy: Dr. Harshith R Rao)

place and the curette is withdrawn followed by introduction of the radial EBUS probe through the guide sheath (EBUS-GS) to reach the site. Once the expected pathology is identified by the radial probe, the curette is then withdrawn. The cytology brush and biopsy needle are then introduced through the guide sheath to obtain specimen sample. While performing radial EBUS using fluoroscopy, the guide sheath is left at position. A metallic ring present in the end of guide sheath acts as a marker. Either biopsy needle and cytology brush are then introduced through the guide sheath under fluoroscopy guidance to arrive at the desired site and obtain specimen sample.

Radial EBUS-GS performed in patients with diagnosis of benign peripheral pulmonary diseases showed better diagnostic accuracy of 58.3% compared to EBUS without GS [1]. Radial EBUS-GS was performed on patients with solitary pulmonary nodules by Xu et al. Using a guide sheath, radial EBUS was able to diagnose solitary pulmonary nodule as malignant in 83.3% cases and as benign lesions in 56.7% cases [2]. In beginners where slim bronchoscope is available the use of guide sheath helped in reducing complications to 1.5% which is the range and the diagnostic yield was also high 73% as studied by Eom et al. [3]. Complications that can occur while performing radial EBUS in peripheral pulmonary lesion using guide sheath was studied by Hayama et al. They found that the overall complications that can occur due to use of guide sheath was 1.3% [4] A study done by Arimura et al. used radial EBUS guide sheath to localize and obtain bronchial brushing, transbronchial biopsy and transbronchial needle aspiration material from the peripheral pulmonary lesion and the diagnostic yield found were 62.9% for bronchial brushing, 80.0% for transbronchial biopsy and 77.1% for transbronchial needle aspiration [5].

A meta-analysis done by Ali et al. [6] on diagnostic yield of radial EBUS for peripheral tumors, found that the diagnostic yield was significantly higher for peripheral lesion >2 cm in size, which were malignant in nature and were associated with a bronchus sign on computerized tomography (CT) scan. They also found that the diagnostic yield was higher when the lesion was around the lumen of the bronchus as compared to the lesion adjacent to it [1]. Meta-analysis done by Lee et al. [7] demonstrated that the diagnostic yield of radial EBUS TBNA without fluoroscopic guidance was found to be 0.70 (95% confidence interval [CI], 0.67–0.74), though there was significant heterogenicity in studies [2].

The pooled diagnostic yield of RP-EBUS-GS-guided transbronchial cryobiopsy (TBCB) without fluoroscopy was 71.5% (103/144). In 133 patients, the diagnostic yield of TBCB was significantly higher than that of transbronchial forceps biopsy (77.4% vs. 59.4%; $P < 0.05$) [8]. The suitability of radial endobronchial ultrasound guided bronchial brushing to add in diagnosis and EGFR genotyping was studied by Yu et al. [9] and found that NSCLC was diagnosed in 66.3% of suspected lung cancer cases and positive cytology report was obtained in 60.3% cases. The diagnostic yield was found to be higher in patients whose chest tomography showed positive bronchus sign and R-EBUS probe located within the lesion [4].

References

1. Zhang L, Wu H, Wang G. Endobronchial ultrasonography using a guide sheath technique for diagnosis of peripheral pulmonary lesions. Endosc Ultrasound. 2017;6(5):292–9. https://doi.org/10.4103/eus.eus_48_17.
2. Xu CH, Yuan Q, Yu LK, Wang W, Lin Y. Endobronchial ultrasound transbronchial biopsy with guide-sheath for the diagnosis of solitary pulmonary nodules. Oncotarget. 2017;8(35):58272–7. https://doi.org/10.18632/oncotarget.16813. Published 2017 Apr 4.
3. Eom JS, Mok JH, Kim I, et al. Radial probe endobronchial ultrasound using a guide sheath for peripheral lung lesions in beginners. BMC Pulm Med. 2018;18(1):137. https://doi.org/10.1186/s12890-018-0704-7. Published 2018 Aug 13.
4. Hayama M, Izumo T, Matsumoto Y, Chavez C, Tsuchida T, Sasada S. Complications with endobronchial ultrasound with a guide sheath for the diagnosis of peripheral pulmonary lesions. Respiration. 2015;90(2):129–35. https://doi.org/10.1159/000431383.
5. Arimura K, Sekine Y, Hiroshima K, et al. The efficacy of transbronchial needle aspiration with endobronchial ultrasonography using a guide sheath for peripheral pulmonary lesions suspected to be lung cancer. Respir Investig. 2017;55(6):365–71. https://doi.org/10.1016/j.resinv.2017.08.004.

6. Ali MS, Trick W, Mba BI, Mohananey D, Sethi J, Musani AI. Radial endobronchial ultrasound for the diagnosis of peripheral pulmonary lesions: a systematic review and meta-analysis. Respirology. 2017;22(3):443–53. https://doi.org/10.1111/resp.12980.
7. Lee J, Song JU. Diagnostic yield of radial probe endobronchial ultrasonography-guided transbronchial biopsy without fluoroscopy in peripheral pulmonary lesions: a systematic review and meta-analysis. Thorac Cancer. 2023;14(2):195–205. https://doi.org/10.1111/1759-7714.14733.
8. Chen H, Yu X, Yu Y, et al. Diagnostic performance of cryobiopsy guided by radial-probe EBUS with a guide sheath for peripheral pulmonary lesions. J Bras Pneumol. 2023;49(1):e20220200. Published 2023 Jan 9. https://doi.org/10.36416/1806-3756/e20220200.
9. Yu KL, Tsai TH, Ho CC, et al. The value of radial endobronchial ultrasound-guided bronchial brushing in peripheral non-squamous non-small cell lung cancer. Sci Rep. 2018;8(1):5837. Published 2018 Apr 11. https://doi.org/10.1038/s41598-018-24300-7.

Indication and Contraindication of EBUS TBNA

8

All interventional and diagnostic procedures are carried out under the purview of defined indications and contraindications. It is therefore required to understand the indications and contraindications of performing EBUS TBNA, for early and better diagnostic yield as well as for patient safety. To enumerate, a few indications and contraindications are listed below for EBUS TBNA.

8.1 Indications

1. The most important indication for EBUS TBNA is evaluation of mediastinal lymph nodes for the diagnosis and staging of lung cancer and administration of appropriate treatment. Contrast enhanced CT thorax and PET scan can demonstrate the size and extent of tumor as well as the metabolic activity respectively but their diagnostic accuracy has been questionable. According to literature, mediastinal lymph node metastasis diagnosis by CECT was found to be have a sensitivity and specificity of 59% (95% CI, 50–67%) and 78%% (95% CI, 70–84%) respectively while PET scan had a sensitivity and specificity of 83% (95% CI, 77–87%) and 92% (95% CI, 89–95%) respectively [1]. Hence, EBUS TBNA is a safer and useful procedure and has better diagnostic yield compared to conventional TBNA. Radial EBUS can also localize mediasti-

M. M. Mohapatra, P. Upadhya, *Handbook of Endobronchial Ultrasound*, https://doi.org/10.1007/978-981-96-0531-6_8

nal lymph nodes and the targeted node can be sampled after removing the probe by inserting appropriate size needle through the working channel of bronchoscope without real time needle monitoring.

2. EBUS is also used for evaluation of benign and granulomatous causes of mediastinal lymphadenopathy. Sarcoidosis and tuberculosis are the granulomatous lymphadenopathy which are evaluated by EBUS TBNA. Other benign and malignant causes of lymph node enlargement like lymphoma are also evaluated when there is dilemma in diagnosis. Some of the mediastinal mass close to the airways are also approached by EBUS for diagnosis.
3. EBUS is used for sampling of solitary peripheral parenchymal pulmonary nodule, endobronchial and peribronchial lesions [2, 3]. Sampling of peripheral pulmonary nodule can be done by bronchoscopy with fluoroscopy guidance. However, radial EBUS probe can be utilized for localization of the peripheral pulmonary tumor and sampling of the lesion without fluoroscopy. The pulmonary lesions can be identified as hypoechoic texture in reference to the surrounding lung tissue and have sharply defined borders due to the interface between aerated lung parenchyma and the lesion. A randomized trial comparing radial probe EBUS sampling with conventional bronchoscopy sampling under fluoroscope guidance showed that the diagnostic yield was 76% and 52% respectively [4]. Lesions which are not visible in fluoroscopy and are less than 3 cm in diameter can also be sampled by radial EBUS.
4. Conventional bronchoscopy can only visualize the airway lumen and the mucosa. EBUS provides an extended view beyond the tracheobronchial wall. The preoperative assessment of airway wall in patients with centrally located tumors for planning of treatment requires to determine the extent of airway wall involvement. EBUS is considered to be an effective diagnostic modality in this case and also can differentiate external compression of the airways from that of tumor infiltration of the airway wall. The inner layers of the airway wall consists of seven layers and as per EBUS the inner two layers are the mucosa and submucosa. The third, fourth and fifth lay-

ers are the cartilage and the external two layers are loose and dense fibroconnective tissue. The external two layers progressively taper and thins out beyond lobar bronchi. Cartilage layers also becomes patchy and finally disappears leaving behind only three layers as we progress to distal airways.

5. In endobronchial obstruction, radial probe EBUS passes through stenosis to determine the patency of the distal airways and longitudinal extent of the tumor. This information helps in planning out interventional procedures by identifying length of stenosis and proximity of any major vessels.
6. EBUS can be used for therapeutic purpose also. It can be used for placement of transbronchial needle injection for malignant tumors and photodynamic therapeutic agents for local recurrence of lung cancer [5, 6]. There are also some reports suggesting the use of EBUS in diagnosis and management of mediastinal bronchogenic cyst [7].
7. EBUS is also helpful for detection of early airway malignancy as it can screen the airway wall and the mucosa.

   Besides lung malignancy detection, mediastinal node staging as well as treatment with curative intent and granulomatous lymphadenopathy aetiologies, EBUS is also helpful in identification of other pathological conditions. These are as follows:

   - EBUS helps in detecting a pulmonary artery mass lesion
   - Linear EBUS can also detect any intracardiac mass lesion
   - Any infected mediastinal cyst can also be well identified for management
   - EBUS can also help in detecting pulmonary embolism in the pulmonary artery
   - It is also helpful for staging of thyroid cancer [8]

8.2 Contraindication

The lists of contraindications is same as that of the normal flexible bronchoscope. It includes patients with cardiac arrhythmias, recent myocardial infarction, heart failure, severe hypoxemia, severe pulmonary hypertension, severe bronchospasm and few relative contraindications like thrombocytopenia, coagulopathy and deranged renal profile [9].

NOTE: Acute coronary syndrome within the previous 4 weeks is an absolute contraindication while performing EBUS-TBNA. This is because EBUS and bronchoscopy can cause hypoxia and hypertension thereby precipitating further myocardial infarction. Patients who have significant coronary disease and have undergone percutaneous coronary procedures in the last year should be carefully planned for EBUS after discussion with the cardiologist. Antiplatelet should be discontinued for at least 5–7 days prior to performing the procedure. Patients those who are on oral anti- coagulant therapy should withhold their medications for 48 h. Those patients who are on warfarin medications and are planned for EBUS procedure should change their medications to other alternative like low molecular weight heparin keeping the international normalized ratio to less than 1.5. If any of the patient are on dual antiplatelet therapy following coronary interventional procedures should be consulted with the cardiologist before performing EBUS procedure.

References

1. Fletcher JW, Djulbegovic B, Soares HP, et al. Recommendations on the use of 18F-FDG PET in oncology. J Nucl Med. 2008;49(3):480–508. https://doi.org/10.2967/jnumed.107.047787.
2. Tyan CC, Machuca T, Czarnecka K, et al. Performance of endobronchial ultrasound-guided transbronchial needle aspiration for the diagnosis of isolated mediastinal and hilar lymphadenopathy. Respiration. 2017;94(5):457–64. https://doi.org/10.1159/000479745.
3. Prasad KT, Muthu V, Sehgal IS, et al. Utility of endobronchial ultrasound-guided transbronchial needle aspiration in HIV-infected patients with undiagnosed intrathoracic lymphadenopathy. Lung India. 2018;35(5):379–83. https://doi.org/10.4103/lungindia.lungindia_480_17.
4. Paone G, Nicastri E, Lucantoni G, et al. Endobronchial ultrasound-driven biopsy in the diagnosis of peripheral lung lesions. Chest. 2005;128(5):3551–7. https://doi.org/10.1378/chest.128.5.3551.
5. Harris K, Oakley E, Bellnier D, Shafirstein G. Endobronchial ultrasound-guidance for interstitial photodynamic therapy of locally advanced lung

cancer-a new interventional concept. J Thorac Dis. 2017;9(8):2613–8. https://doi.org/10.21037/jtd.2017.07.45.

6. Mehta HJ, Jantz MA. Endobronchial ultrasound-guided intratumoral injection of cisplatin for the treatment of isolated mediastinal recurrence of lung cancer. J Vis Exp. 2017(120):54855. Published 2017 Feb 12. https://doi.org/10.3791/54855.
7. Maturu VN, Dhooria S, Agarwal R. Efficacy and safety of transbronchial needle aspiration in diagnosis and treatment of mediastinal bronchogenic cysts: systematic review of case reports. J Bronchol Interv Pulmonol. 2015;22(3):195–203. https://doi.org/10.1097/LBR.0000000000000174.
8. Fantin A, Castaldo N, Tirone C, et al. Endobronchial ultrasound: a pictorial essay. Acta Biomed. 2023;94(4):e2023113. Published 2023 Aug 3. https://doi.org/10.23750/abm.v94i4.14090.
9. Steward M, Dickson C. Sonography endobronchial assessment, protocols, and interpretation. [Updated 2023 Feb 6]. In: StatPearls [Internet]. Treasure Island: StatPearls Publishing; 2023. Available from: https://www.ncbi.nlm.nih.gov/books/NBK570578/.

9 Therapeutic Indications of EBUS

While EBUS has been employed in the diagnosis and assessment of mediastinal lymph nodes and bronchogenic cysts, limited literature is present on therapeutic implications of EBUS. There are few published articles regarding therapeutic use of EBUS in pericardial effusion, and thyroid gland lesions as non-malignant causes where EBUS had been of great use [1]. In malignant lesion EBUS has been of therapeutic use in form of laser resection, argon plasma coagulation, electrosurgery, cryotherapy, brachytherapy, photodynamic therapy, and stenting for intra luminal lesions to relieve symptoms and administer treatment.

9.1 Therapeutic Indications

(a) EBUS is useful as an adjunct to improve the safety of therapeutic procedures. Herth et al. in his study on therapeutic use of endobronchial ultrasound found that EBUS was used before mechanical tumor debridement of central tumors, in airway stenting and before as well as during administering ND: YAG laser and argon plasma coagulation. This effort not only changed the result of therapy but also helped in better guidance of treatment [2].

M. M. Mohapatra, P. Upadhya, *Handbook of Endobronchial Ultrasound*, https://doi.org/10.1007/978-981-96-0531-6_9

(b) EBUS prevented the use of longer stents for endoscopically unappreciated submucosal and parabronchial tumor extension thereby withdrawing the use of this intervention.
(c) EBUS facilitated the precise assessment of tumour penetration through the airway wall and providing a clear visualization of vessels. This enabled the clinicians to halt debridement with laser or APC when approaching critical structures ensuring a more targeted therapeutic approach.
(d) While administering photodynamic therapy (PDT), EBUS provides a more accurate assessment of tumor invasion compared to conventional bronchoscopy and HRCT. As a result tumours which had cartilaginous involvement were better treated with photodynamic therapy thereby avoiding inadvertent use of PDT [3].
(e) In case of mediastinal lymph node metastasis or advanced mediastinal lung cancer, EBUS guided instillation of radioactive agents was found to be effective. Study done by Xu et al. found that installation of EBUS guided interstitial iodine-125 in mediastinal nodes was effective and safe [4].
(f) Cystic lesions in the mediastinum account for approximately 12–18% of all mediastinal lesions in adults. Among these, bronchogenic cysts are the most prevalent, making up to 50% of all mediastinal cysts in the adult population. Endobronchial ultrasound (EBUS) is increasingly being used for the diagnosis of mediastinal lesions using both endosonographic characteristics and cytologic examination of aspirated material. Venkata N Maturu in his systematic review of case reports found that therapeutic aspiration of mediastinal bronchogenic cyst by EBUS not only helped in diagnosis but also was an alternative to surgery [5].
(g) The primary strategies for extending survival and enhancing the quality of life in patients with obstructive, inoperable lung cancer involve tumour debulking and airway recanalization [6]. Endobronchial intra-tumoral chemotherapy is a viable option for patients across all stages of non-small cell lung cancer (NSCLC), spanning from stage I to IV. When dealing with extraluminal diseases such as masses or lymph nodes that induce compressive airway obstruction, it is recom-

mended to insert the needle into the wall at an angle ranging from approximately 60° to 90° [6]. Two case reports where endobronchial ultrasound guided transbronchial needle instillation of chemotherapeutic agents were attempted and resulted it resolution of the tumor in PET scan [6, 7].

(h) Electromagnetic navigated brachytherapy is now being tried as a new treatment option for peripheral pulmonary tumours. The radial EBUS is performed after localization of the tumour and placement of the catheter to confirm the exact position in the central location of the tumour [8].

Endobronchial ultrasound has now routinely used for diagnostic procedures. The use of EBUS in therapeutic intervention and adjunct to other interventional study are now being evaluated and has become an area of interest for research for future directions.

References

1. Mohan A, Madan K, Hadda V, Mittal S, Suri T, Shekh I, et al. Guidelines for endobronchial ultrasound-transbronchial needle aspiration (EBUS-TBNA): Joint Indian Chest Society (ICS)/Indian Association for Bronchology (IAB) recommendations. Lung India. 2023;40(4):368–400.
2. Herth F, Becker HD, LoCicero J, Ernst A. Endobronchial ultrasound in therapeutic bronchoscopy. Eur Respir J. 2002;20(1):118–21.
3. Miyazu Y, Miyazawa T, Kurimoto N, Iwamoto Y, Kanoh K, Kohno N. Endobronchial ultrasonography in the assessment of centrally located early-stage lung cancer before photodynamic therapy. Am J Respir Crit Care Med. 2002;165(6):832–7.
4. Xu T, Peng WD, Gu X, Yu WJ. Endobronchial ultrasound-guided iodine-125 radioactive seed implantation as a novel therapy for mediastinal tumors. Cancer Biother Radiopharm. 2019;34(9):547–50. https://doi.org/10.1089/cbr.2019.2818.
5. Maturu VN, Dhooria S, Agarwal R. Efficacy and safety of transbronchial needle aspiration in diagnosis and treatment of mediastinal bronchogenic cysts: systematic review of case reports. J Bronchol Interv Pulmonol. 2015;22(3):195–203.
6. Li X, Liu X, Rao X, Zhao J, Xu Y, Xie M. A case report of local treatment of inoperable squamous cell lung carcinoma with convex-probe endobronchial ultrasound-guided intratumoral injection of cisplatin in a patient with severe COPD. Medicine (Baltimore). 2017;96(24):e7070.

7. Khan F, Anker CJ, Garrison G, Kinsey CM. Endobronchial ultrasound–guided transbronchial needle injection for local control of recurrent non–small cell lung cancer. Ann Am Thorac Soc. 2015;12(1):101–4.
8. Harms W, Krempien R, Grehn C, Hensley F, Debus J, Becker HD. Electromagnetically navigated brachytherapy as a new treatment option for peripheral pulmonary tumors. Strahlenther Onkol. 2006;182(2):108–11. https://doi.org/10.1007/s00066-006-1503-2.

10 Prerequisite and Preparation

The procedure is preferably done on an outpatient basis by a trained interventional bronchoscopist. The learning curve for a trained bronchoscopist may need at least 10 procedures to perform a proper EBUS TBNA while an untrained bronchoscopist may need 30 procedures. The procedure is carried out in a fully equipped endoscopy room or operation theatre consisting of specialized staff, presence of anaesthesiologist and life-saving equipment.

10.1 Preprocedural Preparation

Preprocedural evaluation in EBUS should be carried out as per American Association of Anaesthesiology guidelines. It is recommended to undergo incentive spirometry prior to the procedure to recruit alveoli and prevent atelectasis. This is particularly required for patients who are obese and have risk of intraprocedural atelectasis.

A pulmonary function test if possible is recommended before posting the patient for endobronchial ultrasound. Always it is advisable to have a recent contrast enhanced CT thorax at hand as the lesion might have undergone change than the previous CT thorax. It will also give an overview about the patient tolerability of the procedure since extensive compression due to intraluminal

M. M. Mohapatra, P. Upadhya, *Handbook of Endobronchial Ultrasound*, https://doi.org/10.1007/978-981-96-0531-6_10

or extraluminal compression of the main bronchus may cause stridor. Patients cardiac condition should also be evaluated with ECG, troponin and if required an NT- pro BNP status.

Preprocedural glucose status along with Hb1ac level is also required along with haemoglobin levels to rule out anaemia. A record of serum electrolyte level prior to procedure for potassium level in patients with end stage chronic kidney disease is also mandatory before posting patients with these comorbidities. Induction of anaesthesia by benzodiazepines and opioids are not routinely done unless patient has anxiety or pain. However, it is best to use propofol and lidocaine for induction of anaesthesia if the bronchoscopist feels the need [1].

EBUS TBNA can be done under conscious moderate sedation or general anaesthesia. As per recommendation, an intravenous catheter and continuous monitoring of vital signs like pulse rate, blood pressure and saturation by pulse oximetry is mandatory via monitors. There must be provision for providing oxygen delivery system by nasal mask, venturi mask or mask with reservoir to maintain a preoxygenation targeted FiO_2 of >0.8. A defibrillator must be at hand with trained personal to manage critical situation. EBUS and its related instruments i.e. light source, processor, integrated bronchoscope and ultrasound monitor should all be placed in one column. Patient's concern and queries has to be addressed before performing the procedure. Patient should also be educated about the procedure that he or she may be undergoing.

There must be either two trained nurse or a bronchoscopy technician with a nurse to perform EBUS. One nurse or the trained technician will be handed the responsibility administer topical lignocaine (2%), clean, prepare the scope and the needles and assist in the procedure. The other nurse will give oral suction, intravenous medications, oxygen and monitor the vitals. The patient should be monitored after the procedure for a period of 1 h if mild sedation has been administered, for 2 h if procedure has been done under deep sedation.

10.2 Anaesthesia in Endobronchial Ultrasound Guided TBNA

The type of anaesthesia and the mode of anaesthesia is an important aspect considered while performing EBUS TBNA. Since ultrasound bronchoscope is thicker in diameter as compared to normal flexible bronchoscope and constant contact with the mucosal wall is required while performing EBUS, the type of anaesthesia used is important as the procedure may take long time. Usually, a moderate anaesthesia is required while performing EBUS but some study recommendations are in favour of general anaesthesia [2, 3]. Mostly propofol, etomidate, ketamine, midazolam, dexmedetomidine and fentanyl are used for this procedure and no neuromuscular blocker are recommended [4]. In case of general anaesthesia, an ETT diameter of 8.5 or 9 mm is preferable. It is preferable to use laryngeal mask or supraglottic airway instead of endotracheal tube for better accessibility and performance of needle aspiration of higher lymph nodes.

References

1. Galway U, Zura A, Khanna S, Wang M, Turan A, Ruetzler K. Anesthetic considerations for bronchoscopic procedures: a narrative review based on the Cleveland Clinic experience. J Thorac Dis. 2019;11(7):3156–70. https://doi.org/10.21037/jtd.2019.07.29.
2. Ciriaco P. Impact of different sedation modalities on endobronchial ultrasound-guided transbronchial needle aspiration (EBUS-TBNA). Mediastinum. 2020;4:20. Published 2020 Sep 30. https://doi.org/10.21037/med-20-22.
3. Agostini L, Facciolongo N, Lusuardi M, et al. Endobronchial ultrasound-guided transbronchial needle aspiration under conscious sedation with meperidine and midazolam. Monaldi Arch Chest Dis. 2017;87(2):768. Published 2017 Jul 18. https://doi.org/10.4081/monaldi.2017.768.
4. Lin TY, Huang YC, Kuo CH, et al. Dexmedetomidine sedation for endobronchial ultrasound-guided transbronchial needle aspiration, a randomised controlled trial. ERJ Open Res. 2020;6(4):00064-2020. Published 2020 Nov 10. https://doi.org/10.1183/23120541.00064-2020.

11 Complications of EBUS TBNA

Over the last decade, endobronchial ultrasound-guided transbronchial needle aspiration (EBUS-TBNA) has become a minimally invasive and highly accurate method for sampling intrathoracic lymph nodes [1]. However, data on complications associated with EBUS-TBNA are not only limited but are also likely to underestimate the true complication rate due to underreporting [2]. The complications of EBUS-TBNA are similar to the complications that occur while performing fibre-optic bronchoscopy.

Various complications, spanning from transient hypoxia to fatalities, have been documented during EBUS-TBNA. Data on complications for EBUS-TBNA were taken from a combination of prospective studies, questionnaire-based studies, and a mix of retrospective studies and case reports. It is imperative that both the proceduralist and the requesting provider are well-informed about the potential complications and device malfunctions associated with EBUS-TBNA. Complications can be infection related, non-infectious or device related. Further to make it more simplified can be divided into common and rare complications (Table 11.1, incidence %) [2–4].

M. M. Mohapatra, P. Upadhya, *Handbook of Endobronchial Ultrasound*, https://doi.org/10.1007/978-981-96-0531-6_11

Table 11.1 Infectious and non-infectious complications of EBUS

Infectious complications	Non-infectious complications	Device related
Pneumonia (0.19%)	Transient hypoxia (5–25%)	Assembly/needle malfunction (0.2–1.3%)
Mediastinitis (0.18%)	Bleeding (especially in patients on antiplatelets/anti-coagulation therapy) (0.68%)	Needle fracture
Mediastinal abscess formation	Pneumothorax (0.03%)	Scope damage
Sepsis (0.01%)		
Fever (variable, 0.5 to 10%)		
Respiratory failure (0.23%)		

Overall, studies have shown that only few factors determine increased complications following EBUS procedure. These are [5]:

- Higher Zubrod score
- Transbronchial lung biopsy

Although no evidence is available to recommend specific interventions to minimize EBUS related complications. Several practical measures can be adopted to enhance safety, as outlined below [2]:

1. Strict adherence to the general principles of asepsis is essential.
2. The stylus and needle must be handled with sterility, particularly when obtaining multiple passes.
3. When introducing or removing the needle into or from the channel, visually confirming the retraction of the needle into the sheath is crucial to prevent scope damage. Proper locking of the needle is essential.

4. For individuals with known asthma, administering a bronchodilator immediately before the procedure can help prevent bronchospasm.
5. Sampling from densely calcified lymph nodes should be avoided to prevent unintentional needle breakage.
6. During needle insertion, excessive force should be avoided, and if necessary, the puncture site should be slightly adjusted.

11.1 Infectious Complications [4–11]

Though EBUS-TBNA is known to be a safe procedure, still an overall low complication rate of 1.4% has been documented even in well-equipped intervention centres. The mechanism of how post procedure infectious complications occurs are as follows:

(a) The entry of oropharyngeal bacteria into the mediastinal compartment can occur while introducing the EBUS scope and needle through the transbronchial passage.
(b) Contamination of the sterile needle may occur while passing through the airways after being ejected from the needle sheath or guide sheath.
(c) The presence of erosion which occurs due to decreased vascularity of a particular area in the lung may be associated with an environment conducive of reduced bacterial clearance and proliferation of infective agents.

    However, few factors are associated with the increased risk of infection while performing the procedures. These risk factors are:

    - Immunosuppression status of the patient
    - Older age group
    - Washing procedure
    - CT thorax showing necrotic node
    - More than recommended number of punctures attempted during TBNA
    - Procedure performed through oesophagus as in EUS

Certain precautions must be followed to avoid infective complications. These include:

- To abstain from concurrent bronchial washings especially high infective groups
- The device needs to be disinfected before every use as per the instructions
- Cardiac patients with prosthetic valves and with infective endocarditis should be dealt with caution. Though there is no recommendation of giving prophylactic antibiotics before performing EBUS-TBNA but in these special cases prophylactic antibiotics may prevent infective complications. However, it is in the discretionary opinion of the treating physician to assess and decide upon administering antibiotics.
- Patients with asplenia who are also at risk of developing infection needs to consider for prophylactic antibiotics to be administered.

Mediastinitis and mediastinal abscess has been reported in literature with a reported incidence of 0.1–0.3%. Clinical vigilance is required for an extended period to observe the symptoms of mediastinitis after the intervention. Mediastinitis symptoms tend to appear after an average period of 18.1 days following the procedure. This occurs when oropharyngeal contents get access to the mediastinal tissues. Surgical procedure to evacuate the abscess and antibiotics to resolve the mediastinitis has to be performed as per literature [12–14].

11.2 Noninfectious Complications

(a) Pneumothorax is also a complication of EBUS procedure and the reported incidence is around 0.03–0.5% [1, 5]. The main risk factors associated with this complication are patients who have emphysematous bullae in their CT thorax or COPD or chronic asthma patients as well as bronchiectasis patients who are not on adequate therapy to control their symptoms of breathlessness and cough. Patients who are administered inadequate sedation and unable to control cough may also have pneumothorax especially while performing radial endobronchial ultrasound. The possible mechanism that are responsible for causing pneumothorax are [15–17]:

- Tracheal micro perforation which might occur due to forceful coughing while performing the endobronchial ultrasound procedure.
- Accidental puncture of an emphysematous bullae which might occur during needle biopsy
- Injury to the lung pleura of a previously unchanged lung pathology
- Spontaneous rupture of an emphysematous bullae which occurs due to an elevated chest pressure resulting from vigorous cough while performing EBUS procedure.
- Ventilation induced barotrauma also called Macklin effect can lead to the breach of mucosa and spread of air to the adjacent tissues through the interconnected fascial planes.

Most of these patients present with acute chest pain, neck, or facial swelling due to pneumomediastinum and dyspnoea with falling oxygen saturation and hypoxia.

Management of this complication varies depending upon the extent of pneumothorax. It may be simple observation with high flow oxygen if the pneumothorax is small or intercostal tube drainage if the pneumothorax is large.

(b) Bleeding is another non infective complication that can occur during performing EBUS procedures. The incidence of this complication ranges from 0.68% to 1.7% as per literature search. The major factors responsible for causing this complication are:

- on anticoagulant treatment and has not reached the desired INR for performing the procedure
- liver disease
- chronic kidney disease with platelet derangement
- bleeding diathesis

Evidence for discontinuing antiplatelets and anti-coagulants prior to EBUS procedure is sparse. Clopidogrel and aspirin both are not associated with increased bleeding risk [18, 19]. Low-dose aspirin can be continued and is advisable to initiate if discontinuing clopidogrel.

- For individuals with cardiac conditions carrying a high thrombosis risk, such as a coronary stent in place, or a prosthetic valve consulting a cardiologist is recommended when considering discontinuation of clopidogrel. Decisions regarding procedures should be made cautiously, weighing the risks and benefits.
- In EBUS transbronchial lung biopsy, deviating from the routine recommended duration for discontinuing anticoagulants does not corelate with a higher risk of clinically significant bleeding. However, specific interventions must be carried out to minimize bleeding complication.

The guidance on discontinuation of antiplatelets and anticoagulants before bronchoscopy is adapted from recommendations for gastro-duodenoscopy and colonoscopy, as outlined in the guidelines of the European Society of Gastrointestinal Endoscopy (ESGE).

A few general measures as useful practice tips can be followed as summarized below [2]:

- Patients undergoing EBUS-TBNA can safely continue aspirin.
- For individuals undergoing EBUS-TBNA, clopidogrel may be continued around the time of the procedure, particularly in cases where the risk of thrombosis is deemed higher than the risk of bleeding.
- Anticoagulants should be stopped before EBUS-TBNA, adhering to the duration recommended for each specific agent.

11.3 Device Malfunctions [20, 21]

Different types of malfunctions can occur in the device itself while performing EBUS procedure. The malfunction can be in the needle or in the endobronchial ultrasound scope. The main causes are enumerated below:

- Assembly/needle malfunction
- Needle fracture
- Scope damage

The incidence of this complication in literature is sparse. However, a study done in Japan by Asano et al. in 455 interventional pulmonology facilities demonstrated that scope damage was 1.33% and needle damage incidence was around 0.2%. The most common site for EBUS scope damage as per their study is the working channel which occurred due to needle perforation of the channel followed by damage to the fibre portion of the scope [6].

Underlying are the few causes of device damage:

- Inadequate sedation or inappropriate use of mouth guard causing patient bite
- Improper placement of the puncture needle in the sheath
- Improper blockage of the puncture needle in the sheath
- Operator inadequate experience
- lymph node calcification
- hitting the bronchial cartilage
- tangential position of the needle requiring more angulation and excessive bending

The incidence of needle and EBUS scope damage can be prevented if few precautions are followed. These are:

- a minimum of 40 procedures should be conducted within a span of at least 2 years to surpass the initial learning curve and attain a satisfactory diagnostic yield in EBUS-TBNA.
- adequate sedation has been administered

- to prevent unintentional needle breakage, it is advisable to refrain from sampling densely calcified lymph nodes.
- during needle insertion, excessive force should be avoided, and if necessary, the puncture site should be slightly adjusted in such situations.
- EBUS needles comprising nitinol has the disadvantage that these needles are resistance to permanent bends and kinks easily.

Even in best hands and appropriate settings, complications can happen following diagnostic EBUS procedures. The most common expected and observed complications are bleeding and cough. Major life-threatening complications include-mediastinitis and tension pneumothorax can also occur in some of the cases. However, some of the complications can be avoided with proper sedation, training, and careful assessment of risk factors to each complication.

References

1. Dhooria S, Sehgal IS, Gupta N, Aggarwal AN, Behera D, Agarwal R. Diagnostic yield and complications of EBUS-TBNA performed under bronchoscopist-directed conscious sedation: single center experience of 1004 subjects. J Bronchol Interv Pulmonol. 2017;24(1):7–14.
2. Mohan A, Madan K, Hadda V, Mittal S, Suri T, Shekh I, et al. Guidelines for endobronchial ultrasound-transbronchial needle aspiration (EBUS-TBNA): Joint Indian Chest Society (ICS)/Indian Association for Bronchology (IAB) recommendations. Lung India. 2023;40(4):368–400.
3. Bellinger C, Dotson T. EBUS-TBNA risks and repairs. Respirology. 2017;22(6):1045–46. https://doi.org/10.1111/resp.13096. Epub 2017 Jun 20. PMID: 28631880.
4. Moon KM, Choi CM, Ji W, Lee JS, Lee SW, Jo KW, et al. Clinical characteristics of and risk factors for fever after endobronchial ultrasound-guided transbronchial needle aspiration: a retrospective study involving 6336 patients. J Clin Med. 2020;9(1):152.
5. Eapen GA, Shah AM, Lei X, Jimenez CA, Morice RC, Yarmus L, et al. American college of chest physicians quality improvement registry, education, and evaluation (AQuIRE) participants. Complications, consequences, and practice patterns of endobronchial ultrasound-guided transbronchial needle aspiration: Results of the AQuIRE registry. Chest.

2013;143(4):1044–53. https://doi.org/10.1378/chest.12-0350. PMID: 23117878; PMCID: PMC3616680.
6. Asano F, Aoe M, Ohsaki Y, Okada Y, Sasada S, Sato S, et al. Complications associated with endobronchial ultrasound-guided transbronchial needle aspiration: a nationwide survey by the Japan Society for Respiratory Endoscopy. Respir Res. 2013;14(1):50.
7. Steinfort DP, Johnson DF, Irving LB. Incidence of bacteraemia following endobronchial ultrasound-guided transbronchial needle aspiration. Eur Respir J. 2010;36(1):28–32. https://doi.org/10.1183/09031936.00151809. Epub 2009 Nov 19. PMID: 19926733.
8. Kang N, Shin SH, Yoo H, Jhun BW, Lee K, Um SW, et al. Infectious complications of EBUS-TBNA: a nested case-control study using 10-year registry data. Lung Cancer. 2021;161:1–8.
9. Serra Mitjà P, Gonçalves Dos Santos Carvalho F, Garcia Olivé I, Sanz Santos J, Jiménez López J, Núñez Ares A, et al. Incidence and risk factors for infectious complications of EBUS-TBNA: prospective multicenter study. Arch Bronconeumol. 2023;59(2):84–9.
10. Punamiya V, Mehta A, Chhajed PN. Bronchoscopic needle aspiration in the diagnosis of mediastinal lymphadenopathy and staging of lung cancer. J Cancer Res Ther. 2010;6(2):134–41.
11. Du Rand IA, et al. British Thoracic Society guidelines on diagnostic flexible bronchoscopy. Thorax. 2001;56(Suppl 1):i1–21.
12. Leong SC, Marshall HM, Bint M, Yang IA, Bowman RV, Fong KM. Mediastinal abscess after endobronchial ultrasound-guided transbronchial needle aspiration: a case report and literature review. J Bronchol Interv Pulmonol. 2013;20(4):338–41.
13. Yokoyama Y, Nakagomi T, Shikata D, Higuchi R, Oyama T, Goto T. Surgical treatment for mediastinal abscess induced by endobronchial ultrasound-guided transbronchial needle aspiration: a case report and literature review. World J Surg Oncol. 2017;15(1):130.
14. Haas AR. Infectious complications from full extension endobronchial ultrasound transbronchial needle aspiration. Eur Respir J. 2009;33(4):935–8.
15. Piroddi IMG, Gatto P, Perazzo A, Barlascini C, Nicolini A. Pneumomediastinum following endobronchial ultrasound– guided transbronchial needle aspiration: a case report. Tanaffos. 2017;16(3):245–7.
16. Gnass M, Szlubowski A, Gil T, Kocoń P, Ziętkiewicz M, Twardowska M, et al. Tension pneumothorax as a severe complication of endobronchial ultrasound-guided transbronchial fine needle aspiration of mediastinal lymph nodes. Kardiochir Torakochirurgia Pol. 2015;12(4):359–62.
17. Boskovic T, Stojanovic M, Stanic J, Pena Karan S, Vujasinovic G, Dragisic D, Zarogoulidis K, Kougioumtzi I, Dryllis G, Kioumis I, Pitsiou G, Machairiotis N, Katsikogiannis N, Papaiwannou A, Madesis A, Diplaris K, Karaiskos T, Zaric B, Branislav P, Zarogoulidis P. Pneumothorax after transbronchial needle biopsy. J Thorac Dis. 2014;6(Suppl 4):S427–34.

https://doi.org/10.3978/j.issn.2072-1439.2014.08.37. PMID: 25337399; PMCID: PMC4203979.
18. Gil HI, Ko RE, Lee K, Um SW, Kim H, Jeong BH. Effects of antithrombotic treatment on bleeding complications of EBUSTBNA. Medicina (Kaunas). 2021;57(2):142.
19. Swiatek K. Antiplatelet exposure and bleeding events in patients undergoing EBUS-TBNA. Int J Respir Pulm Med [Internet]. 2017 [cited 2023 Dec 26];4(3). Available from: https://clinmedjournals.org/articles/ijrpm/international-journal-of-respiratory-and-pulmonary-medicine-ijrpm-4-074.php?jid=ijrpm.
20. Bante N, Singh A, Gupta A, Mittal A, Suri JC. Accidental breakage of needle tip during endobronchial ultrasound-guided transbronchial needle aspiration: A case report and review of literature. Lung India. 2021;38(1):80–3. https://doi.org/10.4103/lungindia.lungindia_537_19. PMID: 33402643; PMCID: PMC8066938.
21. Uchimura K, Yamasaki K, Hirano Y, Sakagami K, Kido T, Mukae H, et al. The successful removal of a broken needle as an unusual complication of endobronchial ultrasound-guided transbronchial needle aspiration (EBUS-TBNA): a case report and literature review. J UOEH. 2019;41(1):35–40.

12 EBUS Staging in Lung Cancer

Lung cancer is a significant cause of cancer-related deaths worldwide. Management of non-small cell lung cancer (NSCLC) depends on the stage. For early stages, treatment is intended as curative with surgical resection and adjuvant therapy. But in advanced stages, it is mainly palliative with a combination of chemoradiation. Therefore, accurately staging the mediastinal lymph nodes before surgery is crucial, as it is not only necessary for providing the correct treatment but also for avoiding unnecessary and invasive procedures like thoracotomy.

There are many diagnostic and staging methods developed to overcome the need of more invasive methods. These methods include mediastinoscopy, surgery (both open and video-assisted thoracoscopic surgery), endobronchial ultrasound-guided needle aspiration (EBUS-TBNA), and endoscopic ultrasound-guided fine needle aspiration (EUS-FNA) [1]. Currently, EBUS-TBNA/EUS-FNA is the preferred method for sampling mediastinal lymph nodes because it is less invasive and provides accurate results [2].

M. M. Mohapatra, P. Upadhya, *Handbook of Endobronchial Ultrasound*, https://doi.org/10.1007/978-981-96-0531-6_12

12.1 Need for Lung Cancer Staging Using EBUS

The staging of non-small cell lung cancer (NSCLC) involves detailing the anatomy and determining the extent of cancer based on the size of the primary tumor (T), regional lymph nodal status (N), and the presence or absence of distant metastasis (M) [3].

The intention of treatment in non-small cell lung cancer (NSCLC) depends on the stage of the disease as either curative with surgery and chemoradiation or palliative with chemotherapy [1, 2]. An essential component of lung cancer staging is determining the extent of mediastinal lymph node involvement [3].

Mediastinal lymph node staging is recommended for patients with potentially resectable non-small cell lung cancer (NSCLC) who meet the following criteria: [4].

- Visibly enlarged mediastinal lymph nodes identified on chest computed tomography (CT).
- Mediastinal lymph nodes showing high standardized uptake value (SUV) on PET-CT.
- Large central airway tumors (>3 cm).
- Individuals diagnosed with adenocarcinoma showing high SUV uptake on PET-CT.

According to international guidelines, following a PET-CT scan, the ideal way to stage mediastinal lymph nodes involves using EBUS-TBNA and/or EUS-FNA.

Additionally, individuals with PET-CT scans showing no signs of N metastasis but having clinical factors indicating a high chance of unexpected N metastasis should also undergo mediastinal staging, like EBUS-TBNA and/or EUS-FNA. This includes cases with PET-CT evidence of N1 disease, tumors larger than 3 cm (T > 3 cm), or tumors located centrally [5].

Using EBUS-TBNA, one can obtain samples from various mediastinal lymph node stations, including paratracheal (levels 2R, 2L, 4R, 4L), subcarinal (level 7), hilar (level 10), interlobar (level 11), and lobar (level 12) lymph nodes. Notably, mediastinoscopy lacks access to the latter three stations. The inclusion of

Esophageal Endoscopic Ultrasound Fine Needle Aspiration (EUS-FNA) broadens the sampling capability to encompass stations 8 and 9 (paraesophageal and pulmonary ligament lymph nodes, respectively) and distant metastatic sites like the liver and the left adrenal gland [6].

12.2 Current Role of Mediastinoscopy in Lung Cancer Staging

- A negative EBUS result doesn't always correspond to a high likelihood of unforeseen N2 disease during surgical resection [7].
- Omitting mediastinoscopy has the potential to reduce additional waiting time, the need for general anaesthesia, and hospitalization.
- Hence, in cases where EBUS-TBNA produces negative results, better approach is to proceed directly to surgery without waiting for confirmation through a second staging procedure like mediastinoscopy.

Disadvantages of Mediastinoscopy

- It can sample only lymph node stations 2L/2R and 4L/4R.
- Requires general anaesthesia
- More procedure and anaesthesia related complications

Various studies comparing the diagnostic yield of EBUS and mediastinoscopy in staging of resectable lung tumors were analyzed. Few studies showed better sensitivity and specificity when both the diagnostic tools were combined while one study suggested there is no statistically significant differences between both the diagnostic modes (Table 12.1).

The invasive methods to diagnose the mediastinal nodes for their staging was carried out. Various studies were analysed to look into which invasive method would be appropriate for which node staging. The anaesthesia used and the complications were also analysed and compared (Table 12.2).

Table 12.1 Summary of studies comparing EBUS and mediastinoscopy in the staging of resectable lung cancer

Author	Study type	Intervention	Results
Sharples et al. (2012) [8]	Prospective open-label, randomized controlled trial (participants were suspected NSCLC with suspected mediastinal node involvement)	Group1: Surgical staging alone Group 2: EBUS followed by surgical staging (if endosonography negative)	EBUS followed by surgical staging; if negative, showed higher sensitivity and negative predictive value
Anname et al. (2010) [9]	Randomized controlled trial (participants were suspected resectable NSCLC with a need for mediastinal staging)	Group1: Surgical staging alone Group 2: EBUS ± EUS followed by surgical staging; if EBUS negative	Phase wise approach combining EBUS and surgical staging showed increased sensitivity and reduced unnecessary thoracotomies compared to surgical staging alone
Bousema et al. (2023) [7]	Randomized controlled trial (suspected resectable NSCLC with a need for mediastinal staging after negative systematic endosonography)	Group 1: Immediate tumor resection Group 2: Mediastinoscopy followed by tumor resection	It suggested avoiding confirmatory mediastinoscopy after negative EBUS TBNA based on the selected noninferiority margin in the rate of unforeseen N2 disease after tumor resection with lymph node dissection
Ernst et al. (2008) RCT [10]	Randomized controlled trial (suspected NSCLC with radiologically enlarged mediastinal lymph nodes	Group 1: Staging by endobronchial ultrasound Group 2: Staging by cervical mediastinoscopy	Endobronchial ultrasound had a higher diagnostic yield compared to mediastinoscopy for sampling of paratracheal and subcarinal nodes
Figueiredo et al. (2020) [11]	Meta-analysis (operable NSCLC with radiologically enlarged mediastinal lymph nodes)	Compared the effectiveness of EBUS-TBNA and mediastinoscopy	No statistically significant difference was observed in sensitivity (81% vs 75%) and specificity (both 100%) between EBUS-TBNA and mediastinoscopy

Table 12.2 Comparison of various invasive diagnostic techniques for mediastinal staging [12, 13]

	Conventional TBNA	EBUS-TBNA	EBUS-TBNA and EUS-FNA	Standard cervical mediastinoscopy
Accessible nodes	2R, 2L, 4R, 4L, 7, 10R, 10L, 11R, 11L	2R, 2L, 3p, 4R, 4L, 7, 10R, 10L, 11R, 11L, 12R, 12L	2R, 2L, 3p, 4R, 4L, 7, 10R, 10L, 11R, 11L, 12R, 12L, left adrenal gland, celiac lymph nodes	2R, 2L, 3, 4R, 4L and 7
Sensitivity	78% (station 2,4,7)	81–89% (station 2,4,7)	86–91%	75–78%
Specificity	100%	100%	100%	100%
Anaesthesia	Under sedation	Under sedation	Under sedation	Under general anaesthesia
Complications	Low (minor bleeding)	Low	Low	High
Issues	No accessibility to aortopulmonary nodes More false negative result	Unreliable access to aortopulmonary nodes	Unreliable access to aortopulmonary nodes	No accessibility to aortopulmonary nodes Lesser accessible stations compared to EBUS-TBNA

12.3 Staging Using EBUS According to Clinical Lung Cancer Stage

(a) Clinical stage N0 or N1 NSCLC:
- For cases with clinical N0 disease, current guidelines do not recommend mediastinal lymph node sampling. However, it is important to note that up to 35% of cases initially deemed as clinical N0 have been pathologically upstaged to pN2.
- A recent meta-analysis, comprising nine studies, found that in the preoperative staging of clinical N0/N1 lung cancer, EBUS demonstrated a pooled sensitivity of 49% (95% CI, 41–57%) and a specificity of 100% (95% CI, 99–100%) [14, 15].
- Considering the potential for upstaging and the limitations of sensitivity in clinical N0/N1 cases, staging by EBUS-TBNA becomes necessary, especially in high-risk patients.

(b) Clinical stage N2 or N3 NSCLC:
- For cases with clinical N2/N3 disease, the recommended treatment options involve a choice between combination chemoradiotherapy or surgery. This applies particularly to those with ipsilateral lymph node metastases.
- A meta-analysis that evaluated the role of EBUS-TBNA in the preliminary assessment of mediastinal staging found that EBUS-TBNA demonstrated a combined sensitivity and specificity of 90% and 99%, respectively. As a result, endosonographic procedures are considered safe and show a high level of accuracy in the initial assessment of the mediastinal stage in NSCLC [16].

(c) Restaging after neoadjuvant chemotherapy in NSCLC:
- It is essential to reevaluate the mediastinal staging in 3A/N2 before moving forward with surgery. The success of surgical outcomes depends on knowing whether mediastinal lymph nodes are involved or not.
- A recent meta-analysis, which included 10 studies involving 574 individuals undergoing mediastinal restaging, utilized EBUS-TBNA and EUS-FNA. The findings showed a

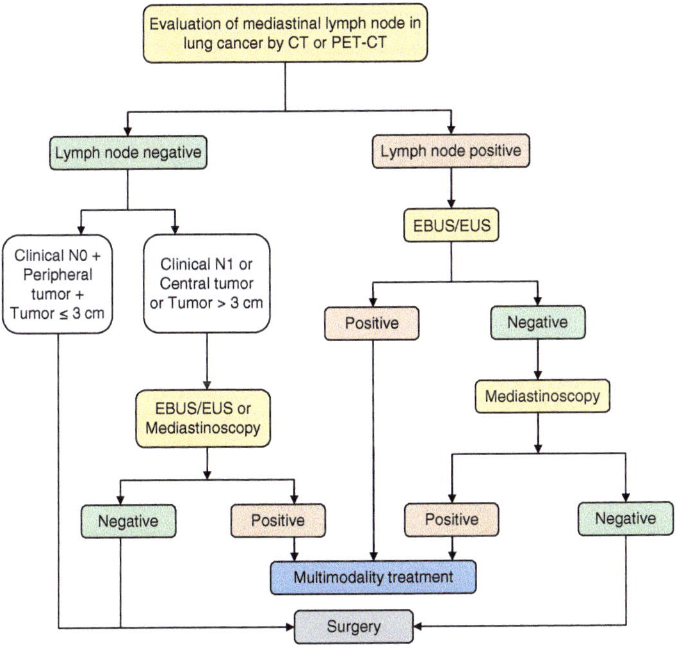

Fig. 12.1 Algorithm for mediastinal staging in lung cancer

combined sensitivity of 67% and a specificity of 99%. Surgical restaging after neoadjuvant therapy can be challenging due to the possibility of mediastinal fibrosis and adhesions [17].

Approach to mediastinal staging in lung cancer patients has been provided in the following algorithm (Fig. 12.1).

12.4 Conclusion

- Endosonographic procedures, particularly endobronchial ultrasound (EBUS), are the preferred primary approach for assessing mediastinal lymph nodes in individuals with clinical stage N0/N1, clinical stage N2/N3, and for mediastinal restaging following neoadjuvant chemotherapy in non-small cell lung cancer (NSCLC).

- Techniques facilitated by endosonography demonstrate heightened sensitivity and specificity, thus enhancing the diagnosis and staging of NSCLC.
- Endosonographic procedures are both safe and reproducible

References

1. Rivera MP, Mehta AC, Wahidi MM. Establishing the diagnosis of lung cancer: diagnosis and management of lung cancer, 3rd ed: American College of Chest Physicians evidence-based clinical practice guidelines. Chest. 2013;143(5 Suppl):e142S–65S.
2. Sehgal IS, Agarwal R, Dhooria S, Prasad KT, Aggarwal AN. Role of EBUS TBNA in staging of lung cancer: a clinician's perspective. J Cytol. 2019;36(1):61–4.
3. Detterbeck FC, Boffa DJ, Kim AW, Tanoue LT. The eighth edition lung cancer stage classification. Chest. 2017;151(1):193–203.
4. Eberhardt WEE, De Ruysscher D, Weder W, Le Péchoux C, De Leyn P, Hoffmann H, et al. 2nd ESMO Consensus Conference in Lung Cancer: locally advanced stage III non-small-cell lung cancer. Ann Oncol. 2015;26(8):1573–88.
5. De Leyn P, Dooms C, Kuzdzal J, Lardinois D, Passlick B, Rami-Porta R, et al. Revised ESTS guidelines for preoperative mediastinal lymph node staging for non-small-cell lung cancer. Eur J Cardiothorac Surg. 2014;45(5):787–98.
6. Yasufuku K, Pierre A, Darling G, de Perrot M, Waddell T, Johnston M, et al. A prospective controlled trial of endobronchial ultrasound-guided transbronchial needle aspiration compared with mediastinoscopy for mediastinal lymph node staging of lung cancer. J Thorac Cardiovasc Surg. 2011;142(6):1393–1400.e1.
7. Bousema JE, Dijkgraaf MGW, van der Heijden EHFM, Verhagen AFTM, Annema JT, van den Broek FJC, et al. Endosonography with or without confirmatory mediastinoscopy for resectable lung cancer: a randomized clinical trial. J Clin Oncol. 2023;41(22):3805–15.
8. Sharples LD, Jackson C, Wheaton E, Griffith G, Annema JT, Dooms C, et al. Clinical effectiveness and cost-effectiveness of endobronchial and endoscopic ultrasound relative to surgical staging in potentially resectable lung cancer: results from the ASTER randomised controlled trial. Health Technol Assess. 2012;16(18):1–75. iii–iv

9. Annema JT, van Meerbeeck JP, Rintoul RC, Dooms C, Deschepper E, Dekkers OM, et al. Mediastinoscopy vs endosonography for mediastinal nodal staging of lung cancer: a randomized trial. JAMA. 2010;304(20):2245–52.
10. Ernst A, Anantham D, Eberhardt R, Krasnik M, Herth FJF. Diagnosis of mediastinal adenopathy-real-time endobronchial ultrasound guided needle aspiration versus mediastinoscopy. J Thorac Oncol. 2008;3(6):577–82.
Figueiredo VR, Cardoso PFG, Jacomelli M, Santos LM, Minata M, Terra RM. EBUS-TBNA versus surgical mediastinoscopy for mediastinal lymph node staging in potentially operable nonsmall cell lung cancer: a systematic review and meta-analysis. J Bras Pneumol. 2020;46(6):e20190221. English, Portuguese. https://doi.org/10.36416/1806-3756/e20190221. Erratum in: J Bras Pneumol. 2021;47(1):e20190221errata. https://doi.org/10.36416/1806-3713/e2019022errata. PMID: 33111752.
11. Sanz-Santos J, Almagro P, Malik K, Martinez-Camblor P, Caro C, Rami-Porta R. Confirmatory mediastinoscopy after negative endobronchial ultrasound-guided transbronchial needle aspiration for mediastinal staging of lung cancer: systematic review and meta-analysis. Ann Am Thorac Soc. 2022;19(9):1581–90.
12. Marshall T, Kalanjeri S, Almeida FA. Lung cancer staging, the established role of bronchoscopy. Curr Opin Pulm Med. 2022;28(1):17–30.
13. Leong TL, Loveland PM, Gorelik A, Irving L, Steinfort DP. Preoperative staging by EBUS in cN0/N1 lung cancer: systematic review and meta-analysis. J Bronchol Interv Pulmonol. 2019;26(3):155–65.
14. Gómez-Caro A, Garcia S, Reguart N, Arguis P, Sanchez M, Gimferrer JM, et al. Incidence of occult mediastinal node involvement in cN0 non-small-cell lung cancer patients after negative uptake of positron emission tomography/computer tomography scan. Eur J Cardiothorac Surg. 2010;37(5):1168–74.
15. Dong X, Qiu X, Liu Q, Jia J. Endobronchial ultrasound-guided transbronchial needle aspiration in the mediastinal staging of non-small cell lung cancer: a meta-analysis. Ann Thorac Surg. 2013;96(4):1502–7.
16. Muthu V, Sehgal IS, Dhooria S, Aggarwal AN, Agarwal R. Efficacy of endosonographic procedures in mediastinal restaging of lung cancer after neoadjuvant therapy: a systematic review and diagnostic accuracy meta-analysis. Chest. 2018;154(1):99–109.

Tips and Tricks: EBUS TBNA 13

The diagnostic yield of EBUS-TBNA is influenced by various factors related to the patient, equipment, and operator. Given its minimally invasive nature and high sensitivity, EBUS-TBNA has become the preferred procedure for staging the mediastinum. Numerous studies have scrutinized different aspects of the EBUS-TBNA process to enhance pathological yield, streamline the procedure, reduce unnecessary steps, and mitigate both time and complications. This chapter aims to provide a comprehensive review of the latest updates concerning the technical performance of EBUS-TBNA and elucidate how emerging data can impact its diagnostic efficacy in conditions such as lung cancer, sarcoidosis, and tuberculosis.

13.1 Choice of Sedation

EBUS-TBNA is typically conducted in the endoscopy suite and is carried out under various levels of sedation, including moderate sedation (MS), deep sedation, or general anaesthesia (GA) [1].

The selection of an anaesthesia strategy for EBUS-TBNA is predominantly influenced by institutional policies and the preferences of the operator.

M. M. Mohapatra, P. Upadhya, *Handbook of Endobronchial Ultrasound*, https://doi.org/10.1007/978-981-96-0531-6_13

EBUS-TBNA tends to be a lengthier procedure compared to flexible bronchoscopy, and the EBUS scope has a larger diameter than its flexible counterpart.

Additionally, EBUS-TBNA involves repeated contact with luminal surfaces.

Therefore, the use of sedation is deemed reasonable to improve patient comfort and minimize coughing during EBUS-TBNA procedures [2].

The type of anaesthesia to be administered to patients undergoing EBUS procedure were also analyzed by study conducted by Casal RF et al. which was a randomized controlled trial where patients were assigned to two groups one with general anaesthesia and the other on moderate sedation. Their study found that the diagnostic yield for EBUS TBNA when done under moderate sedation was comparable to that done under general anaesthesia with 70.7% positivity in the general anaesthesia group and 68.9% in the moderate sedation group with no statistically significant difference with a p value of 0.816. There was no significant difference in rate of complications and patients comfort between the two groups [3].

13.2 Needle Size

There are several commercially available types and sizes of needles for performing EBUS-TBNA, including biopsy needles and TBNA needles. In a meta-analysis conducted by Giri et al. and published in 2015, a comparison between 21-G and 22-G needles were undertaken. The findings revealed no significant difference in diagnostic yield or sample adequacy between the two needle sizes [4]. Another recent meta-analysis compared the diagnostic sensitivities of 19G, 21G, 22G, and 25G needles in lymph nodes suspected for lung cancer. The analysis revealed a high diagnostic yield with overall sensitivities of 93%, 87%, and 85% for 19G, 21G, and 22G needles, respectively [5]. In a recent systematic review and meta-analysis, the impact of needle size on the diagnosis of sarcoidosis was evaluated. The study reported that the

Table 13.1 Comparison of various needle size with their diagnostic yield

Intervention	Patient group/No of participants (n)	Result
Needle size 22G vs. 25G [7]	Lung cancer 102	No statistically significant difference in diagnostic yield
Needle size 22G vs. 19G [8]	Lung cancer 107	No statistically significant difference noted in diagnostic yield. Excessive bloody passes and lower sample adequacy were observed with the 19G needle aspirates
22G and 21G needles [9]	Sarcoidosis 151	21G and 22G were comparable in their diagnostic yield
EchoTip ProCore 22G needle [10]	Sarcoidosis 100	This needle did not demonstrate a superior diagnostic yield than a standard 22G needle

19G needle demonstrated higher sensitivity in comparison to the 21G and 22G needles [6]. Other randomized controlled trials comparing the different needles with their diagnostic yield were compared as mentioned in the below (Table 13.1).

13.3 Use of Suction and Stylet

Traditionally, during EBUS-TBNA, the needle is advanced with a stylet occluding the needle until the lymph node is accessed under EBUS guidance. The purpose of using a stylet during EBUS-TBNA is to prevent airway cells, bronchial wall debris, and blood from entering and filling the inner lumen of the needle, aiming to maintain the quality of the obtained samples. However, the evidence regarding the efficacy of the stylet for this specific purpose remains unclear. The application of suction during EBUS has not been standardized, but its use may enhance the yield by increasing the number of aspirated cells. Number of randomized trials were carried out to find out whether applying suction gives a better yield rather than doing the EBUS procedure without applying any suction to get better retrieval of sample (Table 13.2).

Table 13.2 Comparison of use of suction and stylet with non-suction technique

Serial no.	Study	Type of study	Number of Patients/LN (n)	Overall Findings
1.	Mohan et al. [11]	Prospective, randomized, non-inferiority trial aimed to compare the use of no suction to 10 mL and 20 mL of suction in the context of EBUS-TBNA	323 lymph nodes	
2.	Casal et al. [12]	Prospective randomized trial to compare the use of suction versus no suction in a specific context, likely EBUS-TBNA.	115 patients	No statistically significant difference was noted in diagnostic yield between the groups. However, the use of suction increased the core tissue acquisition rate compared to situations where no suction was applied. There was no significant difference in sample adequacy or diagnostic yield when performing EBUS-TBNA with or without the use of a stylet.
3	Lin et al. [13]	Randomized controlled trial to compare three different techniques during a medical procedure: suction with a stylet, suction without a stylet, and stylet without suction [13].	97 patients	

13.4 Fanning

Fanning is a technique employed by endoscopists to enhance the diagnostic yield of a procedure. It involves sampling multiple areas within a lymph node during each pass by altering the angle of the needle with each subsequent agitation. Studies involving ex vivo calf lungs have demonstrated that using fanning methods during EBUS-TBNA collected larger tissue samples compared to procedures without fanning. This suggests that the fanning technique may contribute to improved specimen size during the sampling process [14].

13.4.1 ProCore Needle

The ProCore® needle from Cook Medical (Bloomington, IN, USA) is specifically designed to offer a histological tissue core, distinguishing it from standard fine needle aspirations that typically yield cytological specimens. This specialized needle is available in two sizes, 22G and 25G, providing flexibility for different clinical requirements.

Two studies were done to demonstrate better diagnostic yield of core needle compared to standard EBUS needle; one study showed that core needle is better while other study did not demonstrate any additional benefit (Table 13.3).

Table 13.3 Comparison of core needle with conventional EBUS needle

Intervention	Type of study, Study group/ no of participants	Study participant	Result
Core needle versus 22G [15]	Retrospective study	235 patients	Core needle biopsy had higher overall sensitivity compared with standard EBUS-TBNA
ProCore versus the standard EBUS-TBNA needle [10]	Randomized controlled trial	100 consecutive patients	This study did not demonstrate a superior diagnostic yield than a standard 22G needle

Currently, there is insufficient evidence to endorse the use of ProCore needle in routine practice. Nevertheless, the decision to utilize the core needle should be based on the operator's competence and the specific context, carefully weighing the patient's safety and associated risk.

13.4.2 Number of Passes

A needle "pass" denotes a discrete insertion and withdrawal of the needle through the airway wall, essentially representing the number of aspirations conducted during EBUS-TBNA at a specific sampling site. The table below shows the number of needles passes attempted while performing EBUS and their diagnostic sensitivity (Table 13.4).

In patients with NSCLC, performing three passes per lymph node station achieves a sample adequacy of nearly 100% and a sensitivity of 95.3%, ensuring high diagnostic accuracy [16].

In patients diagnosed with sarcoidosis, the cumulative yield achieved with four passes per patient—whether obtained from a single lymph node station or distributed as two passes from each of two lymph nodes amounted to 85% [17].

Table 13.4 Comparison of number of passes and their yield while performing EBUS TBNA

Study	Patient group, no of patients (N)	result
Lee et al. (2008) [16]	Non-small cell lung cancer 102 patients	The sensitivity for differentiating malignant from benign LN stations was 69.8%, 83.7%, 95.3%, and 95.3% for one, two, three, and four aspirations, respectively.
Oki et al. (2018) [17]	Stage I/II sarcoidosis 109 patients	The cumulative yields through the first, second, third, fourth, fifth, and sixth passes for the main target lesion were 63, 75, 82, 85, 86 and 88%, respectively.

13.5 Rapid On-Site Evaluation (ROSE)

ROSE of EBUS-TBNA samples enables swift assessment of sample adequacy and provides a preliminary diagnosis before completing the full specimen evaluation. This real-time technique involves the immediate examination of cytological specimens and is typically performed concurrently with sequential sampling during the EBUS-TBNA procedure.

To perform this, a cytological microscope is placed in the procedure room. This approach is valuable for assessing sample adequacy, facilitating triage of samples for ancillary studies, and offering a provisional diagnosis in real-time [18].

Various studies done to evaluate the improved diagnostic yield using ROSE technique while performing EBUS TBNA were also observed (Table 13.5).

Hence, it was concluded that ROSE does not enhance the diagnostic yield of EBUS-TBNA but performing ROSE reduces the number of passes and the requirement of additional bronchoscopy procedures.

Table 13.5 Comparison ROSE technique with yield of EBUS TBNA

Study, year	Type of study	Result
Trisolini et al. (2015) [19]	Randomized trial where consecutive patients with suspected or known advanced lung cancer were randomly assigned to undergo EBUS-TBNA without ROSE (EBUS arm) or with ROSE (ROSE arm).	EBUS-TBNA with ROSE were less likely to have sample inadequacy for molecular testing (0 vs 6, P =0 .05) and were more likely to have the bronchoscopy terminated after a single biopsy site
Madan et al. (2017) [20]	Randomization trial was conducted in a 1:1:1:1 ratio into four groups: conventional transbronchial needle aspiration without ROSE (TBNA-NR), conventional TBNA with ROSE (TBNA-R), EBUS-TBNA without ROSE (EBUS-NR), and EBUS-TBNA with ROSE (EBUS-R).	Conventional TBNA with ROSE and EBUS-TBNA (with or without ROSE) was superior to conventional TBNA alone.

(continued)

Table 13.5 (continued)

Study, year	Type of study	Result
Sehgal et al. (2018) [21]	Meta-analysis Five studies (618 subjects; two EBUS-TBNA, two conventional TBNA, and one both)	Although ROSE neither improved the diagnostic yield nor reduced the procedure time during TBNA, it was associated with fewer number of needle passes during EBUS-TBNA

13.6 Elastography

Elastography is a diagnostic technique that evaluates tissue stiffness and the distribution of stiffness within a selected region by measuring the tissue's response to mechanical stress. In the context of lymph nodes, those infiltrated by malignancy tend to exhibit increased stiffness and reduced deformability compared to normal tissue [22]. Qualitatively, the 3-color pattern classification by Izumo is one of the most commonly described methods for EBUS elastography [22].

The use of elastography and its benefit was studied while performing EBUS TBNA (Table 13.6).

In settings with a higher prevalence of malignancy, elastography may be useful in distinguishing between malignant and benign lymph nodes, demonstrating variable sensitivity (64–100%) and specificity (65–92%). However, it's important to note that there is limited elastography data available from tuberculosis-endemic settings. The Izumo 3-color classification is the most widely used elastography parameter.

An approach to diagnosis of suspected granulomatous mediastinal node needs to be framed in developing countries where tuberculosis burden is quite high (Fig. 13.1).

Table 13.6 Studies evaluating use of elastography in EBUS for malignancy diagnosis

Study, year	Study design	Number of patients/nodes	Result
Korrungruang, (2017) [23]	Prospective observational study conducted on patients referred for the evaluation of intrathoracic lymphadenopathy, lymph nodes (LNs) were qualitatively classified based on elastographic color patterns.	120 patients	EBUS elastography holds promise as a diagnostic modality for distinguishing between benign and malignant lymph nodes during EBUS-guided transbronchial needle aspiration (TBNA).
Roca et al. (2019) [24]	Patients were randomly assigned to two groups: one undergoing endobronchial ultrasound (EBUS) and the other undergoing EBUS-elastography.	100 nodes	Lymph nodes exhibiting a predominantly blue elastographic pattern were found to be associated with a pathological diagnosis of malignancy. The probability of such nodes presenting malignant infiltration with this color pattern was 86.7% ($P = 0.00004$).
Gupta et al. (2019) [25]	Retrospective single-center study, of endobronchial ultrasound (EBUS) scope to assess elastography patterns based on color distribution.	105 nodes	In the context of the study's elastography classification: Type 1 lymph nodes were determined to have benign pathology in 91.30% of cases (42 out of 46) and malignant pathology in 8.70% of cases (4 out of 46). Type 3 nodes were identified as benign in 44.82% of cases (13 out of 29) and malignant in 55.14% of cases (16 out of 29)

(continued)

Table 13.6 (continued)

Study, year	Study design	Number of patients/nodes	Result
Madan et al. (2022) [26]	Prospective study with subjects undergoing Endobronchial Ultrasound-Guided Transbronchial Needle Aspiration (EBUS-TBNA) were enrolled, and elastography features were observed. The study specifically included subjects with a definitive diagnosis of tuberculosis (TB) or sarcoidosis.	96 patients	Ultrasound elastographic characteristics of lymph nodes demonstrate limited diagnostic utility in distinguishing between tuberculosis (TB) and sarcoidosis during Endobronchial Ultrasound-Guided Transbronchial Needle Aspiration (EBUS-TBNA).
Madan et al. (2022) [27]	Meta-analysis	20 studies (1600 patients, 2712 nodes) were selected.	Ultrasound elastography proves valuable in distinguishing between malignant and benign lymph nodes during endobronchial ultrasound-guided transbronchial needle aspiration. Nonetheless, it is important to note that elastography does not replace the necessity for actual lymph node aspiration, which remains a critical component of the diagnostic process

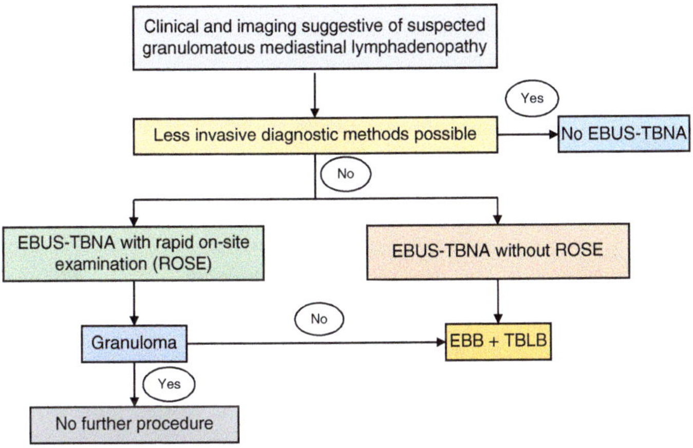

Fig. 13.1 Diagnostic algorithm for suspected granulomatous mediastinal adenopathy in developed countries [28]

To enumerate the various proven methods to increase diagnostic yield of EBUS-TBNA in various conditions, the following table can be referred.

Malignancy including lung cancer and lymphoma	Sarcoidosis	Tuberculosis
More passes (atleast 3/patient) >1 node sampling (atleast 2) Moderate sedation 19G needle (more material especially in lymphoma) Suction (increase core tissue acquisition) Intra nodal forceps biopsy (especially in lymphoma) Elastography (in low tuberculosis endemic area.)	More passes (atleast 4/patient) >1 node sampling (atleast 2 nodes) Sedation Combining with EBB or/and TBLB Cryobiopsy Intranodal forceps biopsy	GeneXpert Culture for drug sensitivity testing

13.7 Summary

Endobronchial ultrasound-guided transbronchial needle aspiration (EBUS-TBNA) continues to be the primary minimally invasive test for assessing mediastinal and hilar adenopathy.

Beyond its role in nodal staging, EBUS-TBNA is valuable for obtaining molecular markers crucial for guiding therapy decisions in patients with non-small cell lung cancer. Additionally, it demonstrates an excellent diagnostic yield, particularly in stages I and II sarcoidosis.

Several factors influence the yield of EBUS-TBNA, including the number of passes, nodes sampled, the level of sedation, operator experience, and the utilization of newer sampling tools such as 19G needles, core needles, and biopsy techniques.

References

1. Canneto B, Ferraroli G, Falezza G, Infante MV. Ideal conditions to perform EBUS-TBNA. J Thorac Dis. 2017;9(Suppl 5):S414–7.
2. Mohan A, Madan K, Hadda V, Mittal S, Suri T, Shekh I, et al. Guidelines for endobronchial ultrasound-transbronchial needle aspiration (EBUS-TBNA): Joint Indian Chest Society (ICS)/Indian Association for Bronchology (IAB) recommendations. Lung India. 2023;40(4):368–400.
3. Casal RF, Lazarus DR, Kuhl K, Nogueras-González G, Perusich S, Green LK, et al. Randomized trial of endobronchial ultrasound-guided transbronchial needle aspiration under general anesthesia versus moderate sedation. Am J Respir Crit Care Med. 2015;191(7):796–803.
4. Giri S, Pathak R, Yarlagadda V, Karmacharya P, Aryal MR, Martin MG. Meta-analysis of 21- versus 22-G aspiration needle during endobronchial ultrasound-guided transbronchial needle aspiration. J Bronchol Interv Pulmonol. 2015;22(2):107–13.
5. Yu Lee-Mateus A, Garcia-Saucedo JC, Abia-Trujillo D, Labarca G, Patel NM, Pascual JM, et al. Comparing diagnostic sensitivity of different needle sizes for lymph nodes suspected of lung cancer in endobronchial ultrasound transbronchial needle aspiration: systematic review and meta-analysis. Clin Respir J. 2021;15(12):1328–36.
6. Kassirian S, Hinton SN, Iansavitchene A, Amjadi K, Chee A, Dhaliwal I, et al. Effect of needle size on diagnosis of sarcoidosis with endobronchial ultrasound-guided transbronchial needle aspiration: systematic review and meta-analysis. Ann Am Thorac Soc. 2022;19(2):279–90.

7. Sakai T, Udagawa H, Kirita K, Nomura S, Itotani R, Tamiya Y, et al. Comparison of the efficiency of endobronchial ultrasound-guided transbronchial needle aspiration using a 22G needle versus 25G needle for the diagnosis of lymph node metastasis in patients with lung cancer: a prospective randomized, crossover study. Translational Lung Cancer Research [Internet]. 2021 [cited 2023 Dec 27];10(9). Available from: https://tlcr.amegroups.org/article/view/56601.
8. Wolters C, Darwiche K, Franzen D, Hager T, Bode-Lesnievska B, Kneuertz PJ, et al. A prospective, randomized trial for the comparison of 19-G and 22-G endobronchial ultrasound-guided transbronchial aspiration needles; introducing a novel end point of sample weight corrected for blood content. Clin Lung Cancer. 2019;20(3):e265–73.
9. Muthu V, Gupta N, Dhooria S, Sehgal IS, Bal A, Aggarwal AN, et al. A prospective, randomized, double-blind trial comparing the diagnostic yield of 21- and 22-gauge aspiration needles for performing endobronchial ultrasound-guided transbronchial needle aspiration in sarcoidosis. Chest. 2016;149(4):1111–3.
10. Dhooria S, Sehgal IS, Prasad KT, Muthu V, Gupta N, Bal A, et al. Diagnostic yield and safety of the ProCore versus the standard EBUS-TBNA needle in subjects with suspected sarcoidosis. Expert Rev Med Devices. 2021;18(2):211–6.
11. Mohan A, Iyer H, Madan K, Hadda V, Mittal S, Tiwari P, et al. A randomized comparison of sample adequacy and diagnostic yield of various suction pressures in EBUS-TBNA. Adv Respir Med. 2021;89(3):268–76.
12. Casal RF, Staerkel GA, Ost D, Almeida FA, Uzbeck MH, Eapen GA, et al. Randomized clinical trial of endobronchial ultrasound needle biopsy with and without aspiration. Chest. 2012;142(3):568–73.
13. Lin X, Ye M, Li Y, Ren J, Lou Q, Li Y, et al. Randomized controlled trial to evaluate the utility of suction and inner-stylet of EBUS-TBNA for mediastinal and hilar lymphadenopathy. BMC Pulm Med. 2018;18(1):192.
14. Parthiban S, Sczaniecka A, Dillard D, Gonzalez X. Comparison of fanning and no-fanning sampling techniques for endobronchial ultrasound-guided transbronchial needle aspiration in an ex vivo tissue model. Chest. 2017;152(4):A964.
15. McCracken DJ, Bailey M, McDermott MT, McManus TE. A retrospective analysis comparing the use of ProCore® with standard fine needle aspiration in endobronchial ultrasound-guided transbronchial needle aspiration (EBUS-TBNA). Ir J Med Sci. 2019;188(1):85–8.
16. Lee HS, Lee GK, Lee HS, Kim MS, Lee JM, Kim HY, et al. Real-time endobronchial ultrasound-guided transbronchial needle aspiration in mediastinal staging of non-small cell lung cancer: how many aspirations per target lymph node station? Chest. 2008;134(2):368–74.
17. Oki M, Saka H, Ando M, Nakashima H, Shiraki A, Murakami Y, et al. How many passes are needed for endobronchial ultrasound-guided trans-

bronchial needle aspiration for sarcoidosis? A prospective multicenter study. Respiration. 2018;95(4):251–7.

18. Li C, Xie W, Cao J, Feng J. Detailed procedure and clinical application overview of rapid on-site evaluation in diagnostic interventional pulmonology. J Res Med Sci. 2020;25:35.
19. Trisolini R, Cancellieri A, Tinelli C, de Biase D, Valentini I, Casadei G, et al. Randomized trial of endobronchial ultrasound-guided transbronchial needle aspiration with and without rapid on-site evaluation for lung cancer genotyping. Chest. 2015;148(6):1430–7.
20. Madan K, Dhungana A, Mohan A, Hadda V, Jain D, Arava S, et al. Conventional transbronchial needle aspiration versus endobronchial ultrasound-guided transbronchial needle aspiration, with or without rapid on-site evaluation, for the diagnosis of sarcoidosis: a randomized controlled trial. J Bronchol Interv Pulmonol. 2017;24(1):48–58.
21. Sehgal IS, Dhooria S, Aggarwal AN, Agarwal R. Impact of rapid on-site cytological evaluation (ROSE) on the diagnostic yield of transbronchial needle aspiration during mediastinal lymph node sampling: systematic review and meta-analysis. Chest. 2018;153(4):929–38.
22. Izumo T, Sasada S, Chavez C, Matsumoto Y, Tsuchida T. Endobronchial ultrasound elastography in the diagnosis of mediastinal and hilar lymph nodes. Jpn J Clin Oncol. 2014;44(10):956–62.
23. Korrungruang P, Boonsarngsuk V. Diagnostic value of endobronchial ultrasound elastography for the differentiation of benign and malignant intrathoracic lymph nodes. Respirology. 2017;22(5):972–7.
24. Hernández Roca M, Pérez Pallarés J, Prieto Merino D, Valdivia Salas MDM, García Solano J, Fernández Álvarez J, et al. Diagnostic value of elastography and endobronchial ultrasound in the study of hilar and mediastinal lymph nodes. J Bronchol Interv Pulmonol. 2019;26(3):184–92.
25. Gupta R, Joshi S, Bhatia A, Tayal N, Pandey P. Qualitative role of endobronchial elastography with endobronchial ultrasound in differentiating malignant and benign lesions: a retrospective single-center study from India. Egypt J Bronchol. 2019;13(5):630–5.
26. Madan M, Mittal S, Tiwari P, Hadda V, Mohan A, Guleria R, et al. The diagnostic utility of ultrasound elastography to differentiate tuberculosis and sarcoidosis during endobronchial ultrasound–guided transbronchial needle aspiration (EBUS-TBNA). Lung India. 2022;39(6):532.
27. Madan K, Madan M, Iyer H, Mittal S, Madan NK, Rathi V, et al. Utility of elastography for differentiating malignant and benign lymph nodes during EBUS-TBNA: a systematic review and meta-analysis. J Bronchol Interv Pulmonol. 2022;29(1):18–33.
28. Prasad KT, Dhooria S, Muthu V, Sehgal IS, Aggarwal AN, Agarwal R. Advantages and drawbacks associated with the use of endosonography in sarcoidosis. Expert Rev Respir Med. 2023;17(4):267–77.

14 Role of EUS and Mediastinoscopy

The mediastinal nodes can be evaluated by both invasive and non-invasive modes. The non-invasive mode of evaluation of mediastinal node can help identify and to certain extent determine the pathology. Since non-invasive mode is not associated with tissue diagnosis it is considered to be inferior compared to invasive mode. The non-invasive mode which are done for evaluation of mediastinal lymph nodes are contrast enhanced computed tomography of thorax (CECT thorax) and positron emission tomography (PET) scan. The invasive mode involves the use of a bronchoscopy. Flexible bronchoscopy can be used to get transbronchial needle aspiration material (TBNA) from enlarged subcarinal node, paratracheal and lower hilar nodes. With the advent of endobronchial ultrasound needle aspiration from other mediastinal nodes became feasible.

Endoscopic ultrasound (EUS) can also be used to obtain guided fine needle aspiration for sampling from mediastinal nodes. The endoscopic ultrasound is introduced into the patient's oesophagus under conscious sedation. It is like that of the EBUS device but thicker in diameter compared to EBUS. EUS also has radial probe and linear probes. EUS is better tolerated by patients than EBUS as there is no coughing or dyspnea symptoms involved in patients.

The function of the radial and linear probe in EUS is same as that of used in EBUS. The radial probe in EUS takes circumferential images or axial view and not recommended for mediastinal

M. M. Mohapatra, P. Upadhya, *Handbook of Endobronchial Ultrasound*, https://doi.org/10.1007/978-981-96-0531-6_14

lymph node biopsy. The linear probe of EUS allows visualization of the mediastinal nodes and has wider view as compared to EBUS. The linear EUS makes an 180° image angle with that of the shaft of the endoscope. A 22gauge needle is passed through the wall of the oesophagus to aspirate material from mediastinal lymph node station 2L, 3A, 4L, 5, 7, 8, 9. EUS can also obtain sample from celiac nodes, left lobe of liver and left adrenal gland [1, 2].

Mediastinoscopy is also used for mediastinal lymph node staging in lung cancer. It can access few of the lymph node stations like 2L, 2R, 4L, 4R, 3 and 7. However, it cannot access lymph node 5, 6, 8 and 9. Its use is hence limited due to its limited access to the mediastinum as well as the cost involved. It has been seen that the estimated cost of both combined EBUS and EUS is less than that of the mediastinoscopy [3].

Mediastinoscope remains an essential tool when EBUS and EUS results are inconclusive. Hence, integration of mediastinoscopy eith EUS and EBUS creates an effective diagnostic triad. This approach helps in comprehensive mediastinal evaluation,diagnostic accuracy and improves patient care in the division of thoracic oncology and mediastinal pathologies.

References

1. Okasha HH, El-Meligui A, Pawlak KM, et al. Practical approach to linear EUS examination of the mediastinum. Endosc Ultrasound. 2021;10(6):406–13. https://doi.org/10.4103/EUS-D-21-00019.
2. Dietrich CF, Annema JT, Clementsen P, Cui XW, Borst MM, Jenssen C. Ultrasound techniques in the evaluation of the mediastinum, part I: endoscopic ultrasound (EUS), endobronchial ultrasound (EBUS) and transcutaneous mediastinal ultrasound (TMUS), introduction into ultrasound techniques. J Thorac Dis. 2015;7(9):E311–25. https://doi.org/10.3978/j.issn.2072-1439.2015.09.40.
3. Navani N, Spiro SG, Janes SM. Mediastinal staging of NSCLC with endoscopic and endobronchial ultrasound. Nat Rev Clin Oncol. 2009;6(5):278–86. https://doi.org/10.1038/nrclinonc.2009.39.

Simulation for EBUS

15

With the growing demand for use of EBUS-TBNA in diagnosis and staging of mediastinal lymph nodes as well as peripheral pulmonary lesion, it is important to undergo simulation-based training that helps in procedural competence. The learning curve of EBUS is variable but it has been suggested that at least 40 to 50 procedures are necessary to have a basic procedural competency [1]. Since training of EBUS-TBNA through clinical encounters can cause increase harm to patients from novice operators, it is advisable to undergo simulation-based training wherever available which will improve learning curve with rapid acquisition of skills. It will improve the knowledge of airway navigation and various procedural skills. Several studies have been done to evaluate the efficacy of simulation-based training compared to conventional training. Konge et al., in his study found that virtual simulation training was more effective than traditional training [2].

Various scores has been assigned for assessment of the initial operator knowledge, behaviour and skills while performing EBUS simulation. EBUSAT, an assessment tool devised to evaluate the competency of initial training curve by using a three-step approach. Step one approach is learning about the anatomy and basic theory of EBUS. Step two is simulation- based training and the third step is supervised practice on patients [2].

M. M. Mohapatra, P. Upadhya, *Handbook of Endobronchial Ultrasound*, https://doi.org/10.1007/978-981-96-0531-6_15

Assessment check lists for assessors are available in form of EBUS Skill and task assessment tool (STAT) or EBUS Skill and Assessment tool (SAT) which are widely available and reproducible for simulation-based method [3]. There are also other tools like step-by-step approach by Bronchoscopy International and web-based curriculum framed by World Association of Bronchoscopy and Interventional Pulmonology. The step-by-step method involves the trainee must first move the bronchoscope to nodal position, obtain a good ultrasound image, set the needle position, aspiration and finally passing the scope through the vocal cords [4].

Since simulation is essential tool in EBUS training, the curriculam needs to be standardized. There is a need for remote simulation platforms and global collaboration for resource sharing and for better professional development. Simulation for EBUS is an important tool for ensuring safety, efficacy and adaptibility to improve diagnostic and therapeutic modality.

References

1. Sehgal IS, et al. Training and proficiency in endobronchial ultrasound-guided transbronchial needle aspiration: a systematic review. Respirology. 2017;22:1547–57.
2. Konge L, Clementsen PF, Ringsted C, Minddal V, Larsen KR, Annema JT. Simulator training for endobronchial ultrasound: a randomised controlled trial. Eur Respir J. 2015;46(4):1140–9. https://doi.org/10.1183/13993003.02352-2015.
3. Bronchoscopy International. (n.d.). Bronchoscopy and Pleural Assessment tools. Retrieved July 2023, from https://bronchoscopy.org/assesssment-tools/.
4. Fielding D. Simulation and assessment tools in EBUS TBNA training: What are we waiting for? Respirology. 2017;22(8):1483–4. https://doi.org/10.1111/resp.13136.

16 Artificial Intelligence and Deep Learning in Endobronchial Ultrasound

Artificial intelligence (AI) is being widely used for interpretation of medical images like chest X-rays, CT scan and MRI and it has been found to improve the diagnosis and classification of diseases. The different types of AI models have been found to have exceeded the expectations of human sciences. AI has few components like machine learning and deep learning which can be used to create models for identifying a disease condition.

Mediastinal lymph node is a difficult site to approach and diagnosing various conditions causing enlargement of these node is important. EBUS is an easier invasive way to approach these nodes. Artificial intelligence is being used in EBUS to understand and differentiate malignant and benign lesions which will be helpful in obtaining a specimen with added accuracy.

Machine learning has the potential to enhance the accuracy and efficacy of endobronchial ultrasound by automated tasking. This system is trained to analyze various EBUS images and classify them into malignant and benign lesions. It also helps in identifying abnormal areas that is not visible to normal eyes by removing noise, improving contrast and improving image quality. Koseoglu et al. found that using artificial neural networks in machine learning models, the machine learning models performed better in differentiating benign from malignant lesion compared to traditional methods [1]. Machine learning computer aided diagnosis (CAD) for prediction of nodal metastasis in lung cancer using endobron-

M. M. Mohapatra, P. Upadhya, *Handbook of Endobronchial Ultrasound*, https://doi.org/10.1007/978-981-96-0531-6_16

chial ultrasound images was studied by Ito et al. and their study showed that CAD based EBUS images had high diagnostic accuracy and specificity and this method can be used to reduce invasive procedure [2]. Patients with stage III NSCLC have regional recurrences at five years after definitive treatment. Identifying of regional lymph node involvement with high sensitivity is required for radiation target volume for tumor control after radiochemotherapy. Guberina et al. used machine learning classifiers to predict nodal involvement and EBUS positivity using PET/CT and histopathology. They demonstrated that PET/CT based machine learning classifiers reduced the misclassification rate compared to standard report. Hence, they suggested that a combined PET/CT based machine learning classifier and EBUS TBNA of PET negative LN station is required to increase sensitivity [3].

EBUS images along with artificial neural networking (ANN) is used for image extraction and textured images to represent and evaluate pixel textural characteristics to identify mediastinal aetiologies are being developed. Ozcelik et al. in his study on artificial neural networking to classify benign and malignant lymph nodes found that ANN could be used along with pixel based information to improve diagnosis accuracy of different lymph node aetiologies [4]. Wang et al. used deep learning algorithms to improve the diagnostic accuracy of mediastinal lymph node sampling using automatic segmentation neural networking of metastatic mediastinal lymph node cytological slides to detect metastasis and help the treating physician to guide further management [5].

Most common EBUS TBNA probe used is the convex probe which is used to derive mediastinal lymph node sample. The sample obtained does not reflect the entire lymph node and hence 20% false negative result is still possible [6]. EBUS convex probe ultrasonographic features can be used to predict the lymph nodes and differentiate between benign and malignant cause. Li et al. in his study validated the deep learning models by comparing with human observation to discriminate automatically benign and malignant lesions with convex probe images [7]. Both unimodal and multimodal deep learning frameworks were developed and validated. This will not only help in proper selection of LN for biopsy and internal puncture site to improve diagnostic efficacy but also help in evaluation of EBUS TBNA in patients with negative results and insufficient tissue volume.

Radial EBUS plays an important role in visualisation and localisation of peripheral lung lesions and improvement in results of transbronchial biopsies. However, some ultrasonic features which are consider to be indicators of malignancy remains unpredictable and depends on the interpretation of the operator. The use of deep learning algorithms to detect lung cancer by ultrasonic image features in radial probe is limited due to artifacts and noise. A multicentre study by Yu et al. studied the feasibility of using convoluted neural networking (CNN) model to differentiate malignant and benign lesion based on radial EBUS images. The dataset was validated internally and externally and the result demonstrated that CNN model can be used as adjunct method for interpretation of radial EBUS sonographic images [8].

Rapid on-site cytological evaluation (ROSE) technique is being applied while performing EBUS for immediate feedback to ensure correct and sufficient sample has been obtained. But this requires a dedicated cytologist to be readily available in the settings. However, very few cytologist perform ROSE as it is time consuming and trained pulmonologist to interpret cytology smears cause interruption of the procedure. Therefore an effective means is required to address these obstacles. Deep learning classification with semantic segmentation model was used by Lin et al. to differentiate whether the smear is from benign or malignant lesion. This study provides future pathways to clinically interpret lung cytology images. In the future, advances in multimodal data integration and AI are expected to address many challanges faced with EBUS. Hence, coordinated work of clinician, engineers and pathologist will help in unlocking the full efficacy of AI and deep learning in EBUS to improve patient outcomes [9].

References

1. Koseoglu FD, Alıcı IO, Er O. Machine learning approaches in the interpretation of endobronchial ultrasound images: a comparative analysis. Surg Endosc. 2023;37:9339–46. https://doi.org/10.1007/s00464-023-10488-x.
2. Ito Y, Nakajima T, Inage T, et al. Prediction of nodal metastasis in lung cancer using deep learning of endobronchial ultrasound images. Cancers (Basel). 2022;14(14):3334. https://doi.org/10.3390/cancers14143334. Published 2022 Jul 8.
3. Guberina M, Herrmann K, Pöttgen C, et al. Prediction of malignant lymph nodes in NSCLC by machine-learning classifiers using EBUS-TBNA and PET/CT. Sci Rep. 2022;12(1):17511. https://doi.org/10.1038/s41598-022-21637-y. Published 2022 Oct 20.
4. Ozcelik N, Ozcelik AE, Bulbul Y, Oztuna F, Ozlu T. Can artificial intelligence distinguish between malignant and benign mediastinal lymph nodes using sonographic features on EBUS images? Curr Med Res Opin. 2020;36(12):2019–24. https://doi.org/10.1080/03007995.2020.1837763.
5. Wang CW, Khalil MA, Lin YJ, Lee YC, Huang TW, Chao TK. Deep learning using endobronchial-ultrasound-guided transbronchial needle aspiration image to improve the overall diagnostic yield of sampling mediastinal lymphadenopathy. Diagnostics (Basel). 2022;12(9):2234. https://doi.org/10.3390/diagnostics12092234. Published 2022 Sep 16.
6. Anantham D, Koh MS, Ernst A. Endobronchial ultrasound. Respir Med. 2009;103(10):1406–14. https://doi.org/10.1016/j.rmed.2009.04.010.
7. Li J, Zhi X, Chen J, et al. Deep learning with convex probe endobronchial ultrasound multimodal imaging: a validated tool for automated intrathoracic lymph nodes diagnosis. Endosc Ultrasound. 2021;10(5):361–71. https://doi.org/10.4103/EUS-D-20-00207.
8. Yu KL, Tseng YS, Yang HC, et al. Deep learning with test-time augmentation for radial endobronchial ultrasound image differentiation: a multicentre verification study. BMJ Open Respir Res. 2023;10(1):e001602. https://doi.org/10.1136/bmjresp-2022-001602.
9. Lin CK, Chang J, Huang CC, Wen YF, Ho CC, Cheng YC. Effectiveness of convolutional neural networks in the interpretation of pulmonary cytologic images in endobronchial ultrasound procedures. Cancer Med. 2021;10(24):9047–57. https://doi.org/10.1002/cam4.4383.

17 Guidelines for EBUS

The **Chest guideline and Expert panel report** in 2016 gave the following evidence based graded recommendation for the technicality of EBUS [1].

- For patients undergoing EBUS-TBNA, either moderate or deep sedation is deemed acceptable (Grade 2C).
- Ultrasonographic features may be utilized to predict malignant and benign diagnoses during EBUS-TBNA; however, it is advised to obtain tissue samples for confirmation (Ungraded Consensus-Based Statement).
- During EBUS-TBNA, tissue sampling can be performed with or without suction (Ungraded Consensus-Based Statement).
- The use of either 21- or 22-gauge needle is recommended as an acceptable option for patients undergoing EBUS-TBNA (Grade 1C).
- In cases where rapid on-site evaluation is unavailable for patients suspected of having lung cancer and undergoing EBUS-TBNA, it is suggested to perform a minimum of 3 separate needle passes per sampling site (Ungraded Consensus-Based Statement).
- For patients undergoing EBUS-TBNA for diagnostic evaluation, it is recommend that tissue sampling can be performed with or without rapid on-site evaluation (Grade 1C).

M. M. Mohapatra, P. Upadhya, *Handbook of Endobronchial Ultrasound*, https://doi.org/10.1007/978-981-96-0531-6_17

- When performing EBUS-TBNA for the diagnosis and/or staging of suspected or known non-small cell lung cancer, it is recommended to obtain additional samples, beyond those needed for the diagnosis, specifically for molecular analysis (Grade 1C).
- During the training EBUS-TBNA operators, it is suggested to incorporate low- or high-fidelity simulation in training process (Grade 2C).
- When assessing EBUS-TBNA operators, it is advisable to employ validated EBUS skills assessment tests for objective evaluation of skill levels (Ungraded Consensus-Based Statement).
- For patients presenting with suspected sarcoidosis and mediastinal and/or hilar adenopathy, the recommended diagnostic approach is the use of EBUS-TBNA (Grade 1C).
- In cases of suspected tuberculosis with mediastinal and/or hilar adenopathy requiring lymph node sampling, the preferred diagnostic method is EBUS-TBNA (Grade 1C).
- For patients suspected of having lymphoma, it is suggested that EBUS-TBNA serves as an acceptable initial and minimally invasive diagnostic test (Ungraded Consensus-Based Statement).

Studies and research are still ongoing to develop robust evidence to provide guidelines for the clinician which needs to be followed while performing EBUS.

The **Joint Indian Chest Society and Indian Association of Bronchology** came up with recommendation for performing EBUS TBNA and this recommendation was prepared based on modified GRADE system [2].

The summary of the recommendation are as follows:

17.1 Antiplatelet and Anticoagulant Therapy and Pre-procedure Coagulation Testing

- It is deemed safe to continue aspirin in patients undergoing EBUS-TBNA (3A)
- In patients undergoing EBUS-TBNA, Clopidogrel may be continued peri-procedurally, especially in cases where the risk of thrombosis outweighs the risk of bleeding (3A)

- Discontinuation of anti-coagulants before EBUS-TBNA is recommended with the duration based on the individual recommendation for each specific agent. (UPP)
- Routine pre-procedure testing for coagulation function and platelet count is not advised among patients undergoing EBUS. (UPP)
- Pre-procedure testing for coagulation function and platelet counts may be considered for patients at high-risk of bleeding including those on anticoagulant therapy, with liver disease, chronic kidney disease, bleeding diathesis, or history of active bleeding. (UPP)

*UPP: Usual Practice Point: defined as important practical points lacking research evidence

17.1.1 Antibiotic Prophylaxis

- The use of prophylactic antibiotics are not recommended for EBUS-TBNA. (2A)

17.1.2 Sedation and Anesthesia

- Administration of sedation is recommended for patients undergoing EBUS-TBNA. (UPP)
- A pre-procedural assessment, utilizing an airway history and a focussed physical examination, should be conducted to anticipate a difficult airway. (UPP)
- EBUS-TBNA should be performed under either moderate sedation or deep sedation/general anaesthesia. (1A)
- The choice between bronchoscopist-directed moderate sedation or anaesthesiologist-directed deep sedation/general anaesthesia is acceptable for EBUS-TBNA. (2B)
- Objective monitoring of the depth of sedation during EBUS-TBNA is recommended and should be conducted by a designated team member. (UPP)

- During EBUS-TBNA under moderate sedation, continuous monitoring of non-invasive blood pressure, oxygen saturation, heart rate and respiratory rate is recommended. (UPP)
- Additional electrocardiographic monitoring is advisable for patients with suspected or known cardiac disease undergoing EBUS-TBNA. (UPP)
- Standard ASA monitoring protocols should be followed as feasible for patients undergoing EBUS-TBNA under deep sedation/general anaesthesia. (UPP)
- Preferably, a combination of sedative agents should be used over a single agent alone, when performing EBUS-TBNA under moderate sedation. (UPP)
- The choice of sedative agent(s) can be determined by operator preference, availability, and monitoring facilities. (UPP)
- When using propofol for sedation, supervision by an anaesthesiologist is preferable. (UPP)
- The supraglottic airway device is the preferred conduit for EBUS-TBNA under general anaesthesia. (2A)
- In patients undergoing EBUS-TBNA under moderate sedation, cricothyroid lignocaine injection may be preferred over spray-as-you-go technique for topical anaesthesia. (1B)
- When utilizing the spray-as-you-go technique, 1% lignocaine is preferred for topical anaesthesia. (1A)

17.1.3 Oxygen Administration

- Routine practice during EBUS-TBNA should involve the suggested to use oxygen supplementation through common oxygen delivery devices such as nasal prongs/nasopharyngeal catheter, coupled with pulse oximetry monitoring. (UPP)

17.1.4 Need for Flexible Bronchoscopic Examination Before EBUS

- At the discretion of the operator, a flexible bronchoscopy for airway assessment may be conducted before the EBUS procedure. (UPP)

17.1.5 Route of Insertion

- The preferred method for EBUS scope insertion is through the oral route. (1A)
- When the oral route is not feasible, using the nasal route for EBUS scope insertion is acceptable if performed by experienced operators. (UPP)

17.1.6 Sonographic Nodal Characteristics and Elastography

- Nodal characteristics identified through endoscopic ultrasound do not serve as a barrier to nodal aspiration for diagnosing mediastinal lymphadenopathy. (3A)
- The use of elastography is not advisable for differentiating malignant from benign mediastinal lymph nodes except for research purposes. (2A)
- EBUS elastography does not eliminate the necessity for tissue sampling. (3A)

17.1.7 Endoscopic Ultrasound with Bronchoscope-Guided Fine Needle Aspiration (EUS-B-FNA)

- EBUS-TBNA is the preferred initial method for sampling accessible mediastinal adenopathy in most patients. (1A)
- In cases where lymph nodes are inaccessible or challenging, the addition of EUS-B-FNA to EBUS-TBNA is recommended for diagnosing malignant nodal involvement and achieving optimal staging in lung cancer. (1A)
- EUS-B-FNA is advised in specific scenarios including lesions inaccessible by EBUS-TBNA, technical challenge with EBUS-TBNA, mediastinal lymph node sampling in pediatric patients, bronchoscopy intolerance, or instances of airway compromise. (3A)
- EUS-B-FNA should be exclusively performed by experienced EBUS operators with dedicated training. (UPP)

17.1.8 Needle Characteristics

- For patients undergoing EBUS-TBNA, it is recommend to use either 21G or 22G needle. (1A)
- The group did not provide any recommendation for or against the use of 19G, 25G, ProCore and Franseen tip needles. The choice of needle is left to the discretion of the operator. (UPP)
- In EBUS-TBNA procedures, it is preferable to use a new needle. (3A)

17.1.9 Use of Suction and Stylet

- EBUS-TBNA can be conducted either with or without the application of vacuum suction. (1A)
- EBUS-TBNA may be performed with or without using a stylet. (1B)
- Stylet maybe used for capillary effect if vacuum suction is not being applied. (UPP)

17.1.10 Use of Balloon Over Ultrasound Probe

- During EBUS-TBNA, it is recommended to routinely attach the balloon. The inflation of the balloon before needle puncture may be carried out based on operator's discretion. (UPP)

17.1.11 Number of Needle Passes

- For all patients undergoing EBUS-TBNA, it is recommended to obtain a minimum of 3 passes per sampled lymph node. (UPP)
- While staging for non-small cell lung cancer (NSCLC) by EBUS-TBNA, it is advisable to perform at least 3 passes per sampled lymph node station. (2A)

- For diagnostic testing and molecular profiling in patients suspected of having lung cancer, a minimum of 4 passes is recommended. (2A)
- In cases of suspected granulomatous mediastinal lymphadenopathy, it is advisable to send additional samples for microbiological molecular analysis. (UPP)

17.1.12 Number of Needle Agitations

- To ensure adequate samples, a minimum of 10 agitation per pass is recommended. (UPP)

17.1.13 Prevention of Complications

- Adhere rigorously to general principles of asepsis. (UPP)
- Handle the stylet and needle in a sterile manner, particularly when obtaining multiple passes. (UPP)
- While introduction and removal of the needle into and from channel, visually confirm the retraction of the needle into sheath to prevent scope damage and ensure proper locking of the needle. (UPP)
- In patients with known asthma, administering a bronchodilator immediately before the procedure may help prevent bronchospasm during the procedure. (UPP)
- To avoid inadvertent needle breakage, refrain from sampling from densely calcified lymph nodes. (UPP)
- Exercise caution to avoid excessive force during needle insertion; if necessary, slightly change the puncture site. (UPP)

17.1.14 Cell Block Preparation

- It is recommended to routinely create cell blocks alongside direct slide smears when obtaining samples during EBUS-TBNA. (2A)

17.1.15 Rapid On-Site Evaluation (ROSE)

- EBUS-TBNA can still be performed regardless of the availability of ROSE. (1A)
- Wherever accessible, it is recommended to perform ROSE during EBUS-TBNA. (2A)
- In situations where ROSE by a pathologist is not feasible, a pulmonologist adequately trained in cytopathology may undertake the ROSE procedure. (3A)

17.1.16 EBUS-TBNA for Non-nodal Pathologies

- Due to high complication rates, it is advisable to refrain from EBUS-guided aspiration of mediastinal bronchogenic cyst. (3B)
- Diagnostic aspiration may be contemplated only when alternative diagnostic methods are either impractical or have proven unsuccessful. (UPP)
- Routine performance of EBUS-guided pericardial fluid aspiration is not recommended. (UPP)
- EBUS-TBNA can be employed for evaluation of intra-thoracic thyroid lesions, especially in situations where percutaneous image-guided needle aspiration is risky and not feasible. (3B)

17.1.17 Endobronchial Ultrasound-Guided Transvascular Needle Aspiration (EBUS-TVNA) and Transbronchial Intravascular Needle Aspiration (EBUS-TIVNA)

- EBUS-TVNA and EBUS-TIVNA may be contemplated only in cases where alternative diagnostic methods are impractical or have proven unsuccessful. (UPP)
- EBUS-TVNA and EBUS-TIVNA should be conducted exclusively by an experienced operator for challenging lesions after

risk-benefit analysis on a case-to-case basis. Patients should undergo close monitoring for potential long-term complications. (3A)

- In all instances of EBUS-TVNA, it is recommended to perform Rapid on-site evaluation (ROSE) to minimize the number of needle passes. (UPP)

17.1.18 Endobronchial Ultrasound-Guided Intra-Nodal Forceps Biopsy (EBUS- IFB)

- EBUS- IFB should be carried out solely by an experienced operator and considered as an additional modality for patients with negative rapid-on-site evaluation (ROSE) or when tissue biopsy is required for definitive diagnosis (e.g. lymphoma). (2B)
- In cases of prior non-diagnostic EBUS-TBNA, the consideration of EBUS-IFB is also warranted. (UPP)

17.1.19 Endobronchial Ultrasound-Guided Mediastinal Cryobiopsy

- Performing EBUS-guided mediastinal cryobiopsy should be reserved for experienced operators and should be applied in situations involving negative rapid-on-site evaluation (ROSE), or prior non-diagnostic EBUS-TBNA. (UPP)

17.1.20 EBUS-TBNA and EUS-B-FNA in Children

Experienced operators can undertake EBUS-TBNA and EUS-B-FNA for sampling mediastinal lymph nodes in paediatric patients. (3A)

- To surmount the initial learning curve and attain an acceptable yield in EBUS- TBNA, a minimum of 40 procedures should be performed over a span of at least 2 years. (2A)

- In the training program for EBUS-TBNA, the incorporation of a virtual reality simulator into the traditional apprenticeship model, wherever feasible. (3B)

  Grading of evidence:

Quality of Evidence	Level
Evidence from >1 well conducted RCT or meta-analysis	1
Evidence from at least 1 moderate quality RCT, or well-designed trial without randomization, or cohort/case control studies	2
Evidence from descriptive studies, reports of expert committees, or opinion of respected authorities based on clinical experience	3
Not backed by sufficient evidence, however, consensus reached by working group based on clinical experience and expertise	UPP
Strength of Recommendations	
Strong recommendation to do (or not to) where the benefits clearly outweigh the risk for most patients	A
Weak recommendation, where the benefits and risks are more closely balanced or are more uncertain	B

References

1. Wahidi MM, Herth F, Yasufuku K, et al. Technical aspects of endobronchial ultrasound-guided transbronchial needle aspiration: chest guideline and expert panel report. Chest. 2016;149(3):816–35. https://doi.org/10.1378/chest.15-1216.
2. Mohan A, Madan K, Hadda V, et al. Guidelines for endobronchial ultrasound-transbronchial needle aspiration (EBUS-TBNA): Joint Indian Chest Society (ICS)/Indian Association for Bronchology (IAB) recommendations. Lung India. 2023;40(4):368–400. https://doi.org/10.4103/lungindia.lungindia_510_22.

Case Studies and Evaluation

1. An 80-year-old female presented with enlarged right lower paratracheal lymph node and was planned for endobronchial ultrasound guided transbronchial needle aspiration (EBUS-TBNA). She was previously admitted with weight loss, haemoptysis and chest pain and was evaluated. Which of the following is a contraindication for performing EBUS on this patient?
   A. Acute exacerbation of COPD 1 month ago
   B. Acute coronary syndrome 2 weeks ago
   C. Angina in last 4 months
   D. Cardiac stenting 2 years ago.
   Answer: B
2. A 56-year-old male, chronic smoker presented to the outpatient clinic with history of loss of weight and appetite and chronic cough for 2 months. He is a known case of type II diabetes mellitus. His contrast enhanced computed tomography of thorax showed a left upper lobe mass lesion with left lower paratracheal lymph node enlargement. His PET CT scan showed suspicious uptake in the left lower paratracheal node. Which is the best modality to stage the suspected lung malignancy?
   A. Perform open mediastinal exploration
   B. Perform EBUS-TBNA of left lower paratracheal lymph node
   C. Perform conventional bronchoscopy transbronchial needle aspiration
   D. Perform CT guided transthoracic needle aspiration
   Answer: B

M. M. Mohapatra, P. Upadhya, *Handbook of Endobronchial Ultrasound*, https://doi.org/10.1007/978-981-96-0531-6

3. A patient presented with history of cough, weight loss and cough and on evaluation his PET CT scan shows right lower paratracheal node enlargement uptake. He was planned for EBUS-TBNA. Which is the ultrasonographic finding that is most specific for metastatic lymph node?
   A. Presence of central hilar sign
   B. Presence of coagulation necrosis
   C. Round distinct margin
   D. Heterogeneous echogenicity.
   Answer: B
4. A 50-year-old female presented with complaints of weight loss, malaise and night sweats. Her computed tomography of thorax shows enlarged mediastinal lymph nodes with uptake on positron emission tomography in stations 3a, 5L and 6L. Which is the most appropriate method to obtain tissue sample in this patient?
   A. Endobronchial ultrasound guided transbronchial needle aspiration
   B. Surgical biopsy through video assisted thoracoscopy
   C. Cervical mediastinoscopy
   D. Endoscopic ultrasound
   Answer: C
5. A patient whose CECT scan shows a right upper lobe mass lesion measuring of about 3.5 × 2.3 cm and has been proven to be adenocarcinoma by CT guided biopsy. CECT thorax of the patient shows enlargement of right lower paratracheal lymph node of size 1.5 cm. What is the best diagnostic modality for staging of the patient before planning of the tumour resection.
   A. Mediastinoscopy
   B. Endobronchial ultrasound- guided transbronchial needle aspiration (EBUS)
   C. Esophageal ultrasound guided fine needle aspiration (EUS)
   D. Combined EUS and EBUS.
   Answer: B

6. As per the Joint Indian Chest Society and Indian Association of Bronchology guidelines, how many passes are required for diagnostic and molecular profiling of lymph node in lung cancer.
   A. 3 passes
   B. 6 passes
   C. 4 passes
   D. 5 passes
   Answer: C
7. What does a guide sheath kit of radial EBUS consists of:
   A. Guide sheath
   B. ET stopper
   C. USG stopper
   D. All of the above
   Answer: D
8. What are the lymph node stations assessed by EUS-B-FNA?
   A. 4L,7,8,9 stations
   B. 4R, 5, 6 stations
   C. 2R, 7, 9 stations
   D. 2L, 5,7, 9 stations
   Answer: A
9. As per recommendation, what is the minimum number of procedures performed required while performing EBUS in paediatric patients?
   A. 30
   B. 50
   C. 40
   D. 60
   Answer: C
10. As per recommendation, should ROSE be performed in EBUS- TVNA after first pass?
   A. To be performed
   B. Not be performed
   C. Depends on the interventionist
   D. TVNA should not be performed
   Answer: A

Test Your Understanding

1. What is the primary application of endobronchial ultrasound (EBUS)?
   (a) Treatment of lung infections
   (b) Minimally invasive evaluation of the mediastinum and lung cancer staging
   (c) Correcting structural defects in the airways
   (d) Performing lung transplants
   Answer: b. Minimally invasive evaluation of the mediastinum and lung cancer staging.
2. What advancements have contributed significantly to the field of thoracic endoscopy?
   (a) Development of pacemakers
   (b) Introduction of new technologies like thin bronchoscopes and EBUS
   (c) Advancements in open chest surgeries
   (d) Development of new antibiotics
   Answer: b. Introduction of new technologies like thin bronchoscopes and EBUS.
3. What are the main indications for using CP-EBUS?
   (a) Treating cardiovascular diseases
   (b) Sampling mediastinal masses and guiding therapeutic interventions
   (c) Performing complex heart surgeries
   (d) Diagnosing neurological disorders
   Answer: b. Sampling mediastinal masses and guiding therapeutic interventions.

M. M. Mohapatra, P. Upadhya, *Handbook of Endobronchial Ultrasound*, https://doi.org/10.1007/978-981-96-0531-6

4. How does elastography assist during endobronchial ultrasound?
   (a) It helps in accelerating the procedure
   (b) By characterizing tissues and informing about their stiffness
   (c) It reduces the need for anesthesia
   (d) By reducing the risk of infection
   Answer: b. By characterizing tissues and informing about their stiffness.
5. CP-EBUS can be used for which of the following?
   (a) Only for sampling lung cancer
   (b) Exclusively for pediatric patients
   (c) Sampling lesions near the airways and for mediastinal disease staging
   (d) Solely for cosmetic procedures
   Answer: c. Sampling lesions near the airways and for mediastinal disease staging.
6. What has been the trend in the detection of lung lesions in recent years?
   (a) Decrease in peripheral lung lesions
   (b) Increase in detection of peripheral lung lesions
   (c) Stable rates of both central and peripheral lung lesions
   (d) Decrease in all types of lung lesions
   Answer: b. Increase in detection of peripheral lung lesions.
7. What impact does the use of RP-EBUS have on lung parenchyma during procedures?
   (a) It leads to the development of atelectasis
   (b) Causes immediate healing of lung tissues
   (c) Reduces lung capacity permanently
   (d) Has no impact on lung parenchyma
   Answer: a. It leads to the development of atelectasis.
8. What are the future research focuses in the field of EBUS technology?
   (a) Focusing solely on pediatric cases
   (b) Reducing the cost of EBUS procedures
   (c) Defining procedural quality endpoints and implementing the technology for therapeutic purposes
   (d) Phasing out EBUS in favor of more invasive procedures
   Answer: c. Defining procedural quality endpoints and implementing the technology for therapeutic purposes.

9. What does the abbreviation 'CP-EBUS' stand for?
   (a) Central Probe—Endobronchial Ultrasound
   (b) Convex Probe—Endobronchial Ultrasound
   (c) Circular Probe—Endobronchial Ultrasound
   (d) Comprehensive Probe—Endobronchial Ultrasound
   Answer: b. Convex Probe—Endobronchial Ultrasound.
10. What is the primary application of elastographic techniques in medical diagnosis?
   (a) Identifying bone fractures
   (b) Tissue characterization
   (c) Blood flow analysis
   (d) Brain activity mapping
   Correct Answer: b. Tissue characterization.
11. Which technique is used in real-time with both transcutaneous and endoscopic ultrasound?
   (a) Shear wave elastography
   (b) Strain elastography
   (c) 3D elastography
   (d) Doppler elastography
   Correct Answer: b. Strain elastography.
12. For what purpose is strain elastography particularly valuable?
   (a) Measuring blood pressure
   (b) Determining bone density
   (c) Discriminating between benign and malignant lymph nodes
   (d) Assessing muscle elasticity
   Correct Answer: c. Discriminating between benign and malignant lymph nodes.
13. What is a potential application of real-time elastography during EBUS?
   (a) Monitoring heart rate
   (b) Selecting lymph nodes for EBUS-guided transbronchial needle aspiration
   (c) Diagnosing neurological disorders
   (d) Performing endoscopic surgery
   Correct Answer: b. Selecting lymph nodes for EBUS-guided transbronchial needle aspiration.

14. Who first described transbronchial needle aspiration (TBNA) for mediastinal lymph node in 1949?
    a) Wang and colleagues
    b) Oho K.
    c) Schieppati
    d) Yasufuku K.
    Correct Answer: c. Schieppati
15. What year marked the development of the convex probe for endobronchial ultrasound?
    (a) 2000
    (b) 2002
    (c) 1998
    (d) 2004
    Correct Answer: b. 2002
16. What is the primary purpose of elastography in the context of EBUS-TBNA?
    (a) To measure tissue oxygenation
    (b) To assess tissue elasticity or stiffness
    (c) To determine the exact size of the lesion
    (d) To visualize the internal structure of the lymph nodes
    Correct Answer: b. To assess tissue elasticity or stiffness
17. Which of the following is a color representation of hard tissue, such as malignancy, in endobronchial elastography?
    (a) Red
    (b) Green
    (c) Blue
    (d) Yellow
    Correct Answer: c. Blue
18. For which of the following lymph node stations is EUS-B FNA particularly useful in lung cancer staging?
    (a) 2R and 4R
    (b) 8 and 9
    (c) 1 and 3
    (d) 5 and 6
    Correct Answer: b. 8 and 9

19. What is the reported accuracy of EBUS in detecting pulmonary embolism (PE)?
    (a) 85%
    (b) 96%
    (c) 75%
    (d) 100%
    Correct Answer: b. 96%
20. What is the role of transvascular needle aspiration (TVNA) in the context of EBUS?
    (a) To improve the visualization of the biopsy site
    (b) To sample lesions behind great vessels
    (c) To diagnose lung cancer
    (d) To assess lung function
    Correct Answer: b. To sample lesions behind great vessels
21. When was Transbronchial Needle Aspiration (TBNA) for mediastinal nodes first described?
    (a) 1983
    (b) 2002
    (c) 1949
    (d) 1978
    Correct answer: c. 1949
22. What is one of the challenges in EBUS-TBNA for molecular analysis?
    (a) High cost of the procedure
    (b) Lack of experienced operators
    (c) Providing a complete molecular analysis
    (d) Difficulty in visualizing the target area
    Correct answer: c. Providing a complete molecular analysis
23. What is the role of Endoscopic Ultrasound with Bronchoscope-guided Fine Needle Aspiration (EUS-B-FNA)?
    (a) To sample lung tissue
    (b) To assist in lung surgeries
    (c) To evaluate lesions not accessible through airways
    (d) To replace traditional bronchoscopy
    Correct answer: c. To evaluate lesions not accessible through airways

24. What is the purpose of endobronchial elastography?
    (a) To measure lung capacity
    (b) To assess the elasticity of lymph nodes
    (c) To evaluate the effectiveness of lung treatments
    (d) To image the trachea
    Correct answer: b. To assess the elasticity of lymph nodes
25. Intratumoral therapy in EBUS is used for?
    (a) Improving diagnosis accuracy
    (b) Delivering drugs directly to tumors
    (c) Monitoring tumor growth
    (d) Providing radiation therapy
    Correct answer: b. Delivering drugs directly to tumors
26. What is a significant advantage of EBUS-guided cryobiopsy?
    (a) Lower cost compared to standard biopsy
    (b) Higher diagnostic yield
    (c) Faster procedure time
    (d) Less invasive than other methods
    Correct answer: b. Higher diagnostic yield

References

1. Fantin A, Castaldo N, Tirone C, et al. Endobronchial ultrasound: a pictorial essay. Acta Biomed. 2023;94(4):e2023113. https://doi.org/10.23750/abm.v94i4.14090. Published 2023 Aug 3.
2. Dietrich CF, Jenssen C, Herth FJ. Endobronchial ultrasound elastography. Endosc Ultrasound. 2016;5(4):233–8. https://doi.org/10.4103/2303-9027.187866.
3. Biondini D, Tinè M, Semenzato U, et al. Clinical applications of Endobronchial Ultrasound (EBUS) scope: challenges and opportunities. Diagnostics (Basel). 2023;13(15):2565. https://doi.org/10.3390/diagnostics13152565. Published 2023 Aug 1.

Annexures

1. Consent form:

Complete details of intended procedure/surgery below:

Both mediastinal and hilar lesions can present in malignant diseases as well as benign disorders. A biopsy specimen for pathological examination is required for diagnosis. Endobronchial ultrasound-guided transbronchial needle aspiration (EBUS-TBNA) biopsy has been widely used for mediastinum lymph node sampling. In this procedure a special type of bronchoscope with a small ultrasound probe in its tip is introduced into the airways. This allows the bronchoscopist to see through the ultrasound the walls of the airways, view lymph glands and blood vessels within the chest cavity. Diagnostic biopsy samples can then be taken from the lymph glands by passing a thin needle through the wall of the airway into the lymph gland. This may not cause too much discomfort. Since the endobronchial ultrasound bronchoscope is wider in diameter than the normal bronchoscope, it is usually introduced through the mouth instead of nose.

Patient Name:
Gender:
Hospital No:
DOB:

M. M. Mohapatra, P. Upadhya, *Handbook of Endobronchial Ultrasound*, https://doi.org/10.1007/978-981-96-0531-6

Health professional statement (To be filled in by health professional with appropriate knowledge of proposed procedure). I have explained the procedure to the patient. In particular I have explained: A. Benefits:

B. Complications are rare but include risk of:

- Infection
- Bleeding
- Pneumothorax
- Pneumothorax following transbronchial biopsy
- Death

Patient's statement: Please read the patient information form carefully. The benefits and risk of the proposed procedure has already been explained to you. Still if you have any further queries regarding your procedure, you are free to ask and we are here to help you. At any point of time, you have changed your mind you are free to withdraw even if you have signed the form.

- I have been explained and understand what the procedure is and why it is being done, including the risks and benefits.
- I agree to the procedure and had the opportunity to ask questions.
- I agree for the use of photography in diagnosis and treatment and for being used for medical teaching and education.
- I understand that any tissue sample removed as part of the procedure may be used for diagnosis, stored or disposed of in a regulated manner by appropriate, ethical, legal and professional standards.
- I understand that any procedure in addition to those described on this form will be carried out only if necessary to save my life or to prevent serious harm to my health.

Name:
Job Title:
Date:
Consultant signature:
Contact details:

Confirmation of consent: On behalf of the team treating the patient, I have confirmed with the patient that they have no further questions and wish the procedure to go ahead.

Consultant Signature:	Patient Signature:

2. Reporting form

ENDOBRONCHIAL ULTRASOUND (EBUS) RECORD

FOB No :- EBUS No:- Date:-
Name: Age / Sex : Ward/OPD :
CR No: CC No : Phone No:
Clinical diagnosis: Operator: Smoking Yes/No:

CXR/CT findings: **Mantoux (in mm):**

Lymph node station	CT Size (long axis)	CT Size (short axis)	USG Size (long axis)	USG Size (short axis)	Passes	Core	No. of Jabbing 10/20	Suction applied 0-20	Stylet used Yes/ No	Visual appearance *L,B,P,BC	Elastography pattern
4R											
4L											
7											
10R											
11R											
10L											
11L											
EUS-B-FNA											
Others (Specify)											

*L- Lymphoid, B- Black, BC – Blood clot, P –Pus

Medication

Atropine+Phenegran	
Midazolam	
Pentazocine/fentanyl	
Ramsay Scale	

EBUS charecteristics of lymph node:

Station	Size (>1cm, >1cm)	Shape(oval, round)	Margin (Disnt/ indsnt)	Echogenicity (HOMO HETERO)/	CHS (Y/N)	CNS (Y/N)	CIV

Clinical parameters

Parameters	Before	During	After

Stain used	
ROSE	
WHOSE cytology	
Cytology on ROSE slide	

Secretions (minimal/copius) – VAS
Cough (minimal/vigorous) – VAS
Procedure duration (mins): EBUS-B-FNA......Needle: Olympus / cook, Size 19G / 21G 22G , Old /New
Complications.........
Aspiration number & report TBNA (final): A.........
Histopath number & report Core: S.........
EBBx: S.........
Cell Block/LBC: A.........
Reason for EUS-B-FNA.........
Final diagnosis.........
COMMENTS.........

Signature

MIX
Papier aus verantwortungsvollen Quellen
Paper from responsible sources
FSC® C105338

If you have any concerns about our products,
you can contact us on
ProductSafety@springernature.com

In case Publisher is established outside the EU,
the EU authorized representative is:
Springer Nature Customer Service Center GmbH
Europaplatz 3, 69115 Heidelberg, Germany

Printed by Libri Plureos GmbH
in Hamburg, Germany